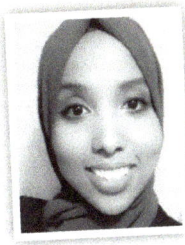

About our Rep, Ayan

Being the only child and raised in a single-parent household as a Muslim, Black African British female in London, Ayan faced many challenges growing up. Like any teenager, Ayan spent this part of life experimenting with the world and what it had to offer her. In search of her identity, she often struggles with "Who am I, what is the purpose of life?".

Ayan's attempt to live a lifestyle more typically associated with western culture was met with rejection and disapproval from her Somali Community. It was not until her lived experience of mental and emotional distress that she embarked on a spiritual journey of self-discovery and personal development, bringing her closer to living her authentic self and rebuilding her faith in Islam.

Ayan has a fascination with wisdom, insight, being genuine, connecting with others without judgement and having deep thoughts. Ayan has chosen to progress her career and personal development by studying her Postgraduate/Masters in Integrative Counselling and coaching. Today, Ayan is fully confident in being a Muslim, British, Black African, Somali female, and she loves the woman she is becoming; full of empathy, compassion, hopes and dreams.

Copyright © 2021 by Emerging Proud Press

All rights reserved. No part of this publication may be reproduced, distributed, or transmitted in any form or by any means, including photocopying, recording, or other electronic or mechanical methods, without the prior written permission of the publisher, except in the case of brief quotations embodied in critical reviews and certain other noncommercial uses permitted by copyright law. For permission requests, write to the publisher, addressed "Attention: Permissions Coordinator," at the address below.

Emerging Proud Press
The Enterprise Centre
Norwich NR4 7TJ
United Kingdom

ISBN: 978-1-7398182-0-3 (paperback)
ISBN: 978-1-7398182-1-0 (e-book)

www.EmergingProud.com

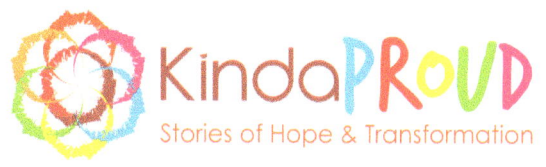

DEDICATION

This book is dedicated especially to Muslims who have been or are going through difficult and painful experiences that are affecting their path through life. Whatever you are going through now, know that these difficult times will end. Know that, this world can be a scary and uncertain place, but we all have the capacity to not just survive but thrive. These stories will demonstrate how this was possible for the Contributors, and so it is all possible for you. Hold on to the hope that someday things for you will be good. No matter what has happened, or how broken you feel, know that you can use this rock bottom as a foundation on which to rebuild your life.

Al Faatiha - The Opener

Chapter One of The Holy Qur'an

In the name of God (Allah), the Most Compassionate, the Most Merciful

All Praises be to God (Allah), Lord of all the worlds

The Most Compassionate, the Most Merciful

Master of the day of judgment

You alone we worship and from you alone, we seek help

Guide us to the straight path

The path of those who have earned your favor, not those who have earned your wrath, nor those who have gone astray.

All stories contained in this Pocket Book are works of memoirs, however, some elements may have been fictionalised. Some names may have been changed to avoid identification. We cannot be held liable for any falsehoods or errors, published by us in good faith, as given to us by the story contributors, including any claims to qualifications, etc. made by story contributors in their personal bios, or religious text or translations used.

We have chosen to keep the stories in the style of each contributor's original submission as much as possible, and native spellings have been used for editing purposes. We have included a Glossary at the back of the book to explain the Islamic terms to support non-Muslim readers' understanding.

The demographics of the storytellers are a natural consequence of who came forward to tell their story and have not been intended as a particular representation, apart from each contributing author identifying as Muslim. We aim to be an inclusive, non-discriminatory project, and we do not align with any one religious or other belief over another.

Any healing modalities, story contributors' personal publications and services, or other resources mentioned within this book are not necessarily endorsed by the team or project. If you are intending to make any significant lifestyle or medication changes as a result of being inspired by reading anyone's story, please seek professional medical advice before doing so.

This project is dedicated to maintaining the integrity of the voices of the people that have shared their stories. The stories shared are real life situations and some of them may contain language that could be triggering for some people, such as suicidal behaviour, violence and upsetting content. We recognise that each individual taking part in the project and reading this book will be at different stages of their transformation journey, and we want to honour that where we're all at is perfectly okay. If you are at all triggered by reading the stories, please seek support from the 'Resources' section in the back of the book.

Praise for this KindaProud Pocket Book

Muslims Emerging Proud through Mental Distress is both a fascinating and empowering collection of experiences.

As we know, trauma can befall anyone, and this incredible book offers hope and inspiration to those experiencing Trauma.

The lived experiences featured in this pocketbook are full of humanity, compassion and determination.

As a Muslim, I resonated with many of the narratives and challenges expressed in this book. I believe this book is essential reading for anyone interested in understanding trauma from a Muslim perspective.

Although awareness surrounding mental health has increased over the years, we still have some way to go regarding the stigma surrounding it. This book will be instrumental in breaking down some of the stigma surrounding mental illnesses, especially within the Muslim community.

I deeply appreciate this book coming into existence and am in awe of the brave individuals that shared their stories.

Zainab Rahman, Founder of Neon Souk

A profound literary piece, brimming with first-hand experiences, genuine stories and poetry filled with bitter sweet moments. Emotional yet elevating, spiritually comforting to the reader, this book is for anybody with an interest in spirituality and discovering ease after hardship. Humanity would benefit from this realistic and practical content.

I enthusiastically recommend this book, as it breaks down many unhelpful stigmas associated with mental health and the Islamic faith. This inspirational book provides endearing, pragmatic advice by uniquely painting the realities of life through the lens of a Muslim that many can relate to.

Sahra Mire, Director of services, Womens Inclusive Team

Three words perfectly describe what you will read in the Muslims Emerging Proud in Mental Distress book:

Beautiful
Powerful
Hopeful

So often, mental health support and resources are full of suggestions without true human authenticity and do not always acknowledge the rawness and pain that comes from trauma and mental distress. Every single story that has been shared in this book is inspiring and perfect, and I feel comforted knowing these words will be shared with others.

The relationship between trauma and mental health is being well established in statutory services and areas of research, particularly since Covid-19 showed itself to the world. However, I always feel like the soul gets forgotten. It is not an added extra, it is the core part of who we are and we cannot ignore it if we are going to talk about pain, distress or how to move beyond being defined by those experiences.

These stories show the importance of caring for our soul and spirituality in an honest, authentic, and profound way.

God lives.

Dr Katie Kelly, Clinical Psychologist & Theology Student

This book is a beautiful collection of powerful stories and poems with extracts from the Qur'an and tips and resources for mental wellbeing. Together these elements weave together to create a holistic book of hope. The authors have really shared from their heart and have shown the importance of having a faith to sustain them.

I hope that the courage of these writers to share their experiences will encourage others to speak out and voice both their struggles and their faith. With service users having a stronger voice and more Experts by Experience working in the NHS, there is increasing opportunity for personal stories such as these to be heard. I was particularly encouraged by the courage of Imran to share his journey as the only male voice in this book. It is a shame that not more men were willing to share their stories. Yet as Imran says there is pressure on men to be strong and yet true strength is when we can be honest with ourselves and with others that we are hurting and need to ask for help. I hope that Imran's strength in sharing his story will encourage other men to find the courage to hold onto their faith as well as to ask for help.

The book also offers a powerful message to those working in mental health services because it highlights the powerful resource that spirituality and faith can be. Too often within NHS settings, people are not treated as whole people and although some recognition is given to the value of spirituality, this needs to be recognised more within mental health provision. Faith can be a powerful source of hope, purpose, resilience and solidarity and when people are facing their toughest moments in life, services need to facilitate, rather than undermine, a person's connection to their faith. Mental health services need to do more to help clients to explore their spirituality at times of crisis and to help those with a faith to see how their beliefs and spiritual resources can be used to sustain them and to facilitate their recovery. The stories in this book are evidence of how faith can help people's health and wellbeing and this is supported by research in this field. (For example, see the Handbook of religion and health (2001) by Koenig, McCullough & Larson which provides a good overview of this research).

Thank you to all those who have contributed to such a wonderful book.

Dr Hilary Garraway, consultant clinical psychologist, former chair of the National Spirituality and Mental Health Forum and BPS

spirituality lead and author of 'Holistic Cognitive Behaviour Therapy', 'Free to be Me' and co-editor of 'Mental Health, Spirituality and Well-being.'
www.hbct.co.uk

Muslims Emerging proud through Mental Distress reveals the individual lived experience of mental distress and how religion can be a source of resilience. This is often a neglected perspective in the understanding of mental distress, which the book addresses in a thoughtful, heartfelt, and reflective way. The book highlights the valuable meaning behind mental distress for Muslims and reveals Islam as a significant strength and resilience. The individual stories give a glimpse into the lifeworld of people who have been through challenging times and found themselves with strength and purpose.

Raisa Kumaga, Director of INAYA Africa Psychological services

No one is listening
They are telling me to wake up
But my eyes are wide open

There's a voice, deep inside me
Whispering…don't let go,
I'm trying to hold on
But I'm slipping away,
I'm hurting and I'm bleeding
Only I can see the blood
Only I can feel the pain
They are pressing on my wounds and I'm screaming,

They don't think I can see them
They think I can't hear them
I'm shouting but my voice has been stolen,
I feel trapped
There's a voice deep inside me
Whispering..please don't let go

Amongst the crowd of them in jackets of white
They look through me
I don't think anyone can see me
But he sees me and she smiles at me
Some can finally hear me
I feel a hand pull me up and I'm standing
I feel pressure on the wound and I stop bleeding,
I'm speaking and one is nodding
My voice, I manage a whisper
I can hear her saying and she reaches out for the oxygen..
We are here for you and we are not letting go…

Sophia

Contents

7	Testimonials
14	About KindaProud
16	Meet the Project's Founder
19	Meet our Peer Pocket Book Rep
28	Peer Stories
128	Resources
132	Self Care Tips
138	Suicidal Thoughts and Self Harm
143	Glossary
147	Acknowledgements
152	The KindaProud Team and other books in the series

About our KindaProud Pocket Book series Ethos and Message

Why do we need Pocket Books of Hope and Transformation? There is a rising epidemic of mental health problems in our society, and alongside it a pervasive negative prognosis message that goes out to those who are struggling emotionally. It's our shared belief, due to our personal experiences, that one of the most important elements of getting back on a road to recovery (and ultimately transformation) is to hear personal stories of HOPE from those who have been there before and not just survived, but thrived.

Each Pocket Book has its own Emerging Proud Rep; a Peer who has personal experience of 'coming through' the theme of that specific book. These are the first 5 books currently in the series:-

- Emerging Proud through NOTEs (Non-Ordinary Transcendent Experiences)

- Emerging Proud through Disordered Eating, Poor Body Image and Low Self-Esteem

- Emerging Proud through Suicide

- Emerging Proud through Trauma and Abuse

- Eye Inspire; #Emerging Proud through Eye Sight Loss

What are the main Aims and Objectives of the KindaProud Pocket Book series?

To relieve people of the distress associated with transformational crises by offering authentic examples of personal stories and resources to engender hope and initiate recovery.

To decrease stigma, improve wellbeing and influence the saving of lives by providing a more compassionate and positive conceptual framework for emotional distress.

To use the profits from book sales to continue to distribute free books, and hence messages of HOPE, to mental health facilities, and those in need, all around the world.

All of the stories in this book have been kindly donated by Muslim Peers who have personally experienced mental and emotional distress and 'emerged transformed' in some way; dedicated to giving hope that there is light at the end of the tunnel to others who may still be suffering. This book series is totally not-for-profit, was seed-funded by *The Missing Kind charity*, and continues to be supported voluntarily through the endless dedication of each peer Rep, and our story contributors.

Meet the Project's Founder

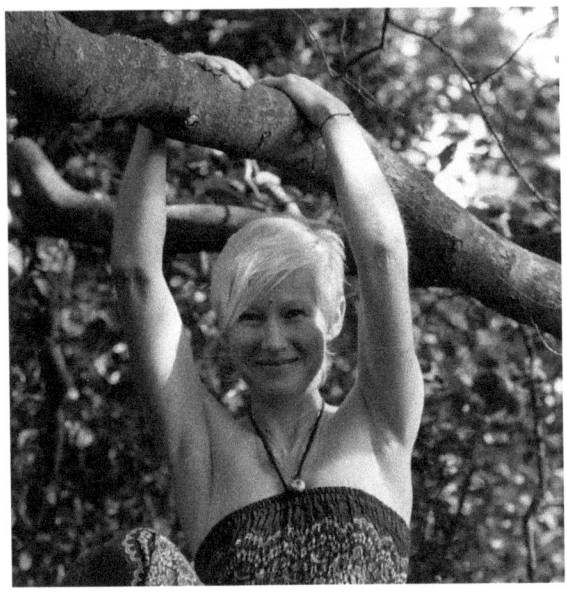

My name is Katie Mottram and I'm the Founder of the Emerging Proud campaign, through which the KindaProud book series has been birthed. Emerging Proud is a grassroots social movement aimed at: 'Re-framing mental distress as a possible catalyst for positive transformation'; providing a platform for people who have 'emerged transformed' through a personal crisis and feel called to share their story and give hope to others.

I was called to start this movement due to finding that re-framing my own crisis as a transformational growth process (which still continues), and hearing the experiences of others, was the thing that helped me to connect with my authentic Self, and start to live the life I was born to live.

When I experienced a personal crisis in 2008, what I needed was a message of HOPE, that all would be okay, not that there was anything 'wrong' with me. I needed to connect with others who had been through similar challenges and were able to walk alongside me whilst I found my own way out of the darkness.

In the last decade, it has been through my own research; looking at more empowering ways of understanding what happened to me, my reactions to it, and how to go about self-healing, in addition to connecting with my amazing peers and listening to their stories, that has really set me on my own path of transformation. This feels like the complete opposite of what I had been told was helpful whilst working within mental health services for 15 years previously. Hence my passion to provide others with the tools that helped me not only to survive, but to thrive and love life.

You can read my full story in my own book, *Mend the Gap: A transformative journey from deep despair to spiritual awakening*, which I published in 2014.

I truly hope that this book, and the others in the 'Pocket Books of Hope and Transformation' series, inspires and supports you in your own evolutionary journey...

And, remember: let that light you hold deep inside shine unapologetically bright - we were ALL born to shine our light in the world - in whatever way that feels right to you!

Find out more about the campaign and what we're up to at: **www.emergingproud.com**

Meet our Peer Pocket Book Rep, Ayan…

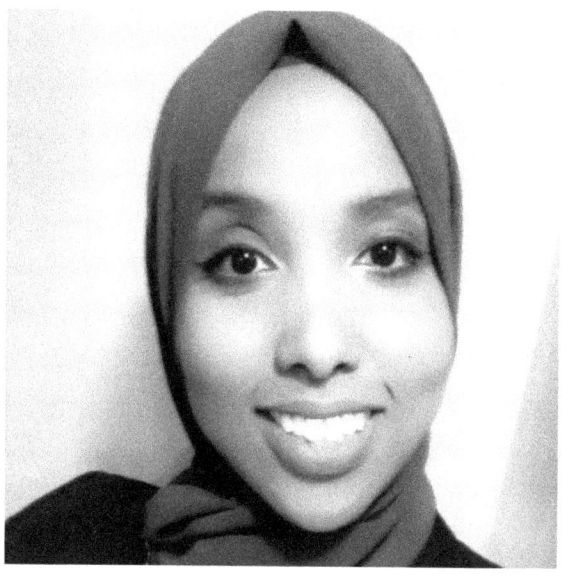

We are so excited to have the inspirational Ayan Hussein to spearhead our special 6th Pocket Book.

Like anyone who has been through a challenging personal journey and found their more authentic Self as a result, Ayan learned that speaking openly about her distress in a safe space, where she could feel heard and validated enough to make sense of her emotions, was the key to her transformation. Ayan has found her purpose through her pain to support others to speak out and have their distress normalised…

I suffered…

During the first few months of being a mother, I remember feeling different within myself. I was often feeling sad for long periods of time.

I looked in the mirror and realised that I didn't know who I was anymore.

I let myself go physically, emotionally and mentally.

I was on autopilot, going through the motions and doing what I had to do as a mother.

Despite this, I would always force a smile in front of others. After all, I didn't want anyone to judge me on my parenting and see me as a 'weak' person. I would constantly feel tearful and hopeless despite having this 'happy mask' on display for others. I was often feeling suicidal, not really to end my life but rather to end my pain.

I recall a day when a family member was talking about mothers that experience symptoms of postnatal depression and the baby blues. I remember thinking that's exactly how I was feeling. No sooner had I convinced myself I was depressed, than another family member declared, "We are Muslims and we shouldn't feel depressed, it is not in our culture or religion".

The day after my eldest was born, a lump appeared in my throat. After a year of many medical tests, the doctors confirmed the lump was a benign tumor, but shortly after I began to experience breathing difficulties. After several hospital visits and further tests it was becoming increasingly clear that the doctors were no further forward in understanding my symptoms.

At that moment my family decided that Ruqya treatment, a form of exorcism in Islam practiced by a Raqi (spiritual healer), might be the answer. Ruqya in Islam is the recitation of the Quran, remembrance and supplications, all used as a means of treating sickness.

My first experience of Ruqya was not a true representation of Islam. Unfortunately, the Raqi abused his power. Spiritual leaders/healers are in a position of trust. It was during this time I was feeling extremely vulnerable and my family turned to this person for support. It was clear he was exerting control over my family, for personal aims and financial gains. This Raqi willfully electrocuted my hands while he recited the Quranic verses, under the false pretence of destroying the bad entity that was inside me.

Things took a turn for the worst; I was not able to eat or sleep for two weeks and I began to feel extremely tormented inside. During this period, I experienced several moments involving the apparent perception of something not present to others, which included seeing visions of strange looking people and hearing voices. These moments became worse at night, which made it almost impossible for me to sleep. I also became extremely paranoid of everyone around me, including my own family. I was taken to the nearest Accident & Emergency Centre and my symptoms intensified. During this period, I was in a complete state of shock to the point where I was muted for a few days.

It didn't end there, I suffered from a major breakdown in my mental wellbeing again after the birth of my second daughter, two years after my first experience of severe mental distress. Yet again my family got worried when I started to get the same symptoms and decided to call a Raqi.

Once again I became extremely ill straight after the session with the Raqi and my family again took me straight to A&E. My symptoms were so intense to the degree that I believed the hospital staff was sent to capture me. Therefore I became suspicious of their actions.

This led me to become both physically and verbally violent and I was sectioned under the Mental Health Act.

I was taken to the Goodmayes psychiatric hospital. I can recall at one point staff members were trying to restrain me. An extreme feeling of fear took over me and I was desperate to get away. There are no words to describe what this experience was like. For some, this matter may seem unimaginable, however only someone who has had this experience might relate. I was eventually given an injection and it knocked me out.

Approximately 2 days later, I had a better awareness of my surroundings and I couldn't comprehend why I was in hospital among people that seemed very unwell.

Eventually, I was moved to a mother and baby unit and this admission marked the beginning of my recovery journey.

Little did I know, when I began this journey, how difficult it was going to be.

Throughout the years, I faced struggles and inner feelings of anger, bitterness, confusion, rejection, and denial. I guess this was due to stigma, which includes self-stigma, lack of acceptance, and lack of knowledge and understanding of mental and emotional distress. I found myself constantly dwelling on the past and projecting it into the future. I frequently experienced flashbacks of the spiritual abuse I suffered.

The turning point was when the urge I had to take responsibility for my life was becoming increasingly irresistible.

I learned...

I have been on a journey of discovery, searching and exploring for different approaches that could aid me in becoming a more emotionally healthy individual. As part of this journey, I have completed a Diploma in counselling skills, an emotional health mentoring course and volunteered for various mental health organisations that focus on improving people's lives. This marked the beginning of my journey of self-research and personal development.

I was part of a research project called ENRICH as a peer worker, which was conducted within the East London Foundation Trust. The 3 years working as a peer worker for ENRICH, where everyone from the project manager, peer coordinators, researchers and the peer workers all had lived experience. This was the most incredible life-changing experience. During this time, I was fortunate to be able to articulate my lived experience and make sense of it.

The most rewarding lesson I learned from ENRICH was the concept of boundaries, both professionally and personally. Setting boundaries based on values that are important to me helps me live a truer life to my authentic self.

For the first time I felt validated, I felt heard, I found clarification to my distress. Healing happens in restoring our lives, sharing our stories in a safe space, without feeling judged or being labeled as our symptoms.

I've managed to recognise some of my painful traumatic events and incidents from childhood that I had suppressed for many years. I learned not to ignore these feelings and emotions, which makes me feel empowered and strong. I also learned how to help someone else go through it.

I have turned my pain into purpose.

The biggest thing that I've realised is that my childhood, my life journey so far and my diverse good and bad experiences - all of these things that I used to think defined me - actually don't define me. *Living in the here-and-now defines me. I can only thank Allah (God) for this journey of inner peace and contentment.*

> **"God (Allah) is the best of planners."**
> Qur'an Surah Ali'Imran, 3:54

However that does not mean I do not sometimes struggle with my emotions or get overwhelmed. I have now gained the tools and techniques that help me bounce back to reality and support me in being emotionally healthier.

Other methods that have assisted me include CBT therapy, Ruqya from a qualified Raqi, and a variety of workshops that cover personal and spiritual development. I undertook counselling with a Muslim counsellor who enabled me to understand what I was going through. I feel that understanding is the key to recovery, the more I learned about my situation the less I feared it.

Taking a holistic approach rather than focusing on one type of method, for example, religious practices have supported me hugely.

Having a great support network also aids one's recovery journey.

When emotional distress enters a family, the emotional cost can be high and family members can be deeply affected. My family is incredibly supportive, I wouldn't be writing my story if it weren't for their continuous support. I believe they have embarked on this journey with me and therefore individually changed for the better.

I changed...

The recovery journey is unique and a continuous one of learning and growing and I'm still on that journey. My lived experience of emotional distress has been extremely hard and bitter, but I am closer to being my authentic self than I ever have been, which is rewarding!

I love the woman I'm becoming, full of empathy, compassion, hopes and dreams.

Everything happens for a reason. There's a hidden blessing behind every complication.

I can accept everything even more because my lived experience has led me to where I am now.

The Islamic concepts of *Qadr* (Divine decree), *tawakkul* (trust in Allah) and *sabr* (patience and forbearance) are finally falling into my body, mind and soul.

I can now accept that life is perfectly imperfect.

I have found my greater sense of purpose, which is helping an individual who may be struggling with any type of emotional distress, no matter what background they come from. As well as my spiritual purpose, which my Lord has explained in His book

> *"And I did not create the Jinn and Mankind except to worship Me"*
> Qur'an Surah Ad-Dhaariyat, 51:56

I suffered. I learned. I changed

Ruphsana emerges proudly with her 'Sisters Story' about how she turned her life around through reframing her experiences

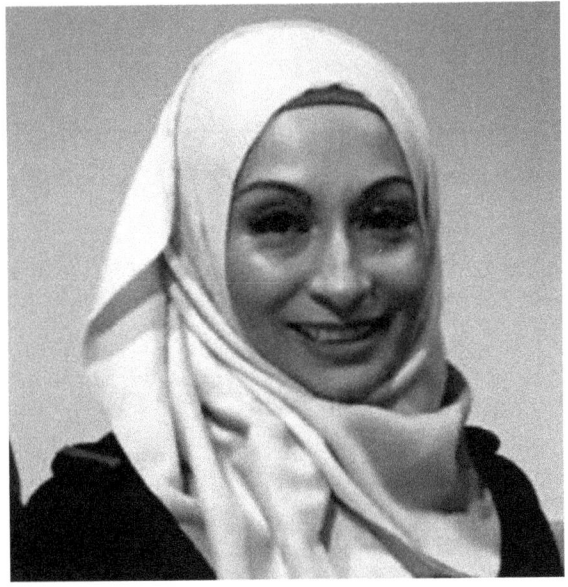

When Ruphsana started to look within she was able to discover the puzzle pieces which enabled her to reframe her story and live life to the full rather than just 'exist' as she had for so many years. Here she proudly emerges to tell all...

"Never underestimate the power of a woman, the love of a mother for her baby or the ability of a woman who has suffered to support other women"
Diane Flores

My Lived Experience with OCD, bulimia, anxiety and postnatal depression, before, during and after my perinatal period:

Today I stand in myself reconnected and whole and yet I am fully aware that my recovery is not a final destination, it will remain an ongoing journey. I would never have imagined that married life was going to take me on a profound journey of losing myself, re-discovering myself and developing a deeper level of self-awareness and spiritual connection to Allah through the whole process. Because of those enriching experiences I now use them to offer other women my hand of hope to help them in their moments of crisis through the perinatal mental health services and by working closely with Approachable Parenting; a community-based organisation that works locally and nationally with families.

I have always been an introspective person as far back as I can remember, very connected to myself; my hopes, my dreams, my values and what my purpose is in life. I grew up with a lot of questions and was never happy to just accept answers that made no sense. These questions were driven by a sense of not belonging. I am the past, present and the future of my existence and I carry the experiences of my parents, who escaped from a war-torn country back in the late 60's/early 70's. I did not 'belong' to my own community because I did not look like them and behave like them. I could not fit into the large south Asian community of largely Pakistani people because I was looked down upon due to my Bangladeshi heritage. I have always been a neat, orderly, fastidious person but not someone who had OCD. I was drawn to harmony, balance and the aesthetic details that stood out from the ordinary.

Condensing down 13 years of struggling - undiagnosed with OCD, intrusive thoughts, anxiety, postnatal depression - I have recently started to talk about my challenging battles with my past addictions with shopping and bulimia around and after my perinatal period. Struggling with my mental health crowded my heart, it ate away all my energy and my ability to think and imagine a different life whilst it chronically imposed upon my peace. There are many reasons why I struggled; guilt, not feeling good enough, fear and judgement from others, my child being taken off me and the lack of information on support services available. And with no diagnosis and no help I continued to silently struggle for many years. For me, the most significant thing was becoming alienated from myself and my own feelings.

After these 13 years of silently struggling I suddenly lost my mother due to ill health. Grief and loss were imposing and demanded to be felt. And for the first time something as drastic as loss rendered me choice-less, I HAD to face my life no matter how painful it was to look. The dark place that I was caught up in opened up to me as a cul-de-sac to my life; that perhaps I could turn around and face a different direction. I started to look at the possibility of "what if I reframe and learn to tell a different story?" and "is it possible to live rather than to just exist?" These possibilities opened my mind and I started to listen to podcasts and learnt new ideas and concepts that gave me hope. Despite my grief, I kept persevering to unlearn the 'faulty thinking' that got me to the place I was in. My recovery was like a jigsaw puzzle with pieces lost along the way and the more I searched, the more I kept finding the pieces, and the bigger picture started to form. Mindfulness or 'khushoo' as I prefer, helped me connect to myself again. The process of change meant radically accepting who I am, my truth, my voice and to face my life and be comfortably still in myself without wanting to run away and hide from the pain. Practicing mindfulness gave me permission to just start again. Finding my 'way' in recovery led to my freedom. Running gave me time to get out and create distance between me and my anxieties. From it I learnt to think about the possibilities of volunteering and helping others. I made a lasting network of new friends who are family to me.

My experiences have taught me to step away from anything extreme and anything that disturbs my peace. I watch and observe potential triggers: for example, I will not weigh, measure or count calories because that will activate those past familiar obsessions. Where once I was trying to find balance and aesthetics in what I consumed and how I looked, I try to live a lifestyle that FEELS GOOD; balanced, permanent and concrete instead of quick fixes that encourage haste and impatience. I have learnt who

I am today and I embrace the good and the not so good aspects of all my life. Turning 40 means getting old enough to look back and join the dots and realize that it was not about finding the jigsaw pieces 'out there', it was about taking a difficult journey inward and connecting it all up together to form My Story today. This is why for me it is non-negotiable when it comes to my peace of mind and my sound heart and not letting anything or anyone disturb it.

"As-Salaam - The Source of Peace"
Name and attribute of God (Allah)

Once a walking contradiction, now Suhur lives with a passion and purpose to help others

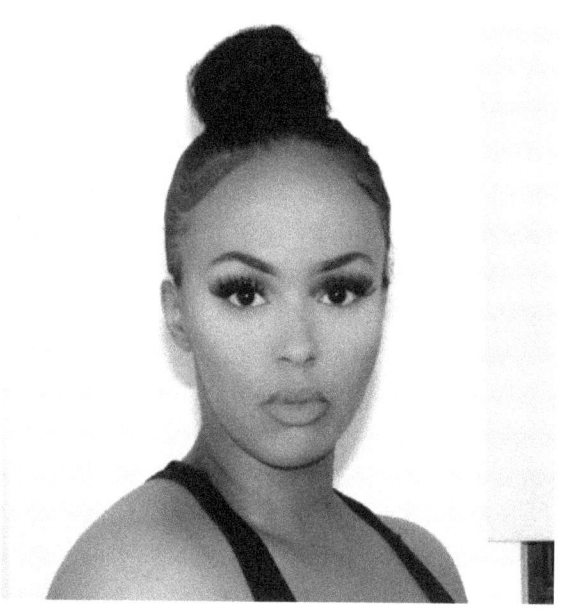

It took a brush with the possibility of losing her life for Suhur to realise that she needed to stop hiding her truth behind a facade of perfection and become the mother to her own hurting inner child. Now Suhur reflects back on this painful time in her life as a blessing, as it was the push she needed to change the way she was seeing herself. Whether you choose to share Suhur's belief that this was God's work or not doesn't really matter, what matters is that when we dare to let down our guard and face our deepest, darkest parts of ourselves, as Suhur was brave enough to do, that is where the magic happens…

It took me a long time to come to a conclusion that Islam as a religion is pure but us as Muslims have faults and are imperfect, especially when we mix religion with culture.

As a 23-year-old Somali Muslim woman I have always known there is a lot of stigma and discrimination towards people with mental and emotional distress.

I think that we live in a culture that values strength and perseverance and has this very naive belief that everyone is born in the same circumstances with the same bodies and the same brains that work the way they're supposed to work.

The challenges British Muslims with mental distress face within the community is stigma and labelling, disrespect and being ignored and the accusations of not being a good practising Muslim. Also the barriers people from Muslim and Somali – African backgrounds face is the lack of mental health literacy, culture of silence (particularly amongst men) and also fear and negative speculation about mental health services and systems.

The stigma is the biggest challenge.

Though labelling and stigma attached to people with emotional distress is rather common among other societies too, it is more intense and more evident in communities that hold the kinship network in high regard. In a nutshell, people with mental distress are stigmatised and accused of being incurable. Distress is seen as being precipitated by individuals not being good practising Muslims. Their families are also stigmatised and accused of not raising their children properly and in Islamic ways. People with emotional issues are ignored by the mainstream community members and they are not talked to, assuming that they are worthless, and their talk is nonsense and a waste of time.

I myself suffered from depression, suicidal thoughts and anxiety. I constantly felt like a walking contradiction. I had dreams and goals that I wanted to achieve and lots of amazing ideas and plans bursting to come out of me, but I felt stuck and blocked. I couldn't consistently act on the things I knew would benefit me and the pressure around it all gave me crippling anxiety which slowed me down further. These patterns developed into a guilt so heavy, it made me dislike myself. Disliking yourself is like hell on earth and the worst way to go through life.

There would be days I would close the blinds, get a duvet, snuggle up on the sofa or my bed and just look up at the ceiling and wouldn't move for days. Other days I would be super productive, and nothing could hold me down.

Nobody knew and, to this day, some people don't know that that girl who had a full face of make-up on and a smile on her face the size of a watermelon was broken deep down inside.

I found myself constantly questioning my purpose and what it was that I was brought into this world to do because I've always known it was nothing average.

I attempted to take my own life in 2017; I remember being in the ambulance with the sirens on, racing to the hospital and it raining so heavily. Through the raindrops on the roof of the ambulance I could hear the paramedic saying to my friend as I came in and out of consciousness "Her heart rate is very high" and "she could die" but I didn't. I am alive for a reason. A purpose. I arrived at the hospital and had my stomach flushed of all the pills I had tried overdosing on. I remember the nurses coming in and saying, "you beautiful girl, why on earth would you do this" and "it will all be okay", all whilst stroking my hair as I looked blankly up at the ceiling avoiding eye contact at all costs.

In the Quran rain is one of the most important factors for life on the earth. Rain carries great importance for all living things including human beings and is a Barakah (a Blessing).

This was my sign. This experience was a blessing. Only lessons and a stronger version of myself was to come from this.

I find such beauty now in being completely broken and rebuilding yourself and that is what kept me going. It was so hard, but I've learned it's all about mastering the balance; you are bound to wobble but it's how you regain that position that matters.

I truly believe Allah (God) has a plan, is the best of planners and only tests the ones he loves the most.

I've never wanted to boast about my suffering in life because there is always somebody who has it worse. I've never wanted sympathy, just for people to try to understand what I am signifying and learn from it. Mental pain can appear less dramatic than physical pain, but it is more common and can also be harder to bear. The frequent attempt to conceal mental pain increases the burden.

It is time we change the mindset around mental health.

I hope to continue pushing for mental health to be a part of schools' curriculums and educate young people.

I hope to bring together communities for discussions on this topic and organise events around mental health.

I always knew I would be great from a young age, but I just didn't know how: now I know it is through helping others by sharing my own experience and breaking this stigma.

Here is a little message to you…

The same month of my suicide attempt, exactly a year later, I had a beautiful daughter and life has been just phenomenal.

Being willing to meet the darkest and deepest part of yourself without any judgement or harshness and being the maternal mother for your inner broken child that the world stepped on is the only way to heal. Giving yourself all the love and light you are desperately seeking outwardly is the only way to heal. The willingness to change the way you see yourself, self-love and putting yourself first is the only way to heal; crying over the old you and welcoming the new you is the only way to heal.

Never give power to the things that broke you or WHO broke you.

Don't be afraid to step forward and be a better you.

"Al Baa'ith - The Restorer of Life"
Name and attribute of God (Allah)

Sophia learned to love herself through her traumatic past

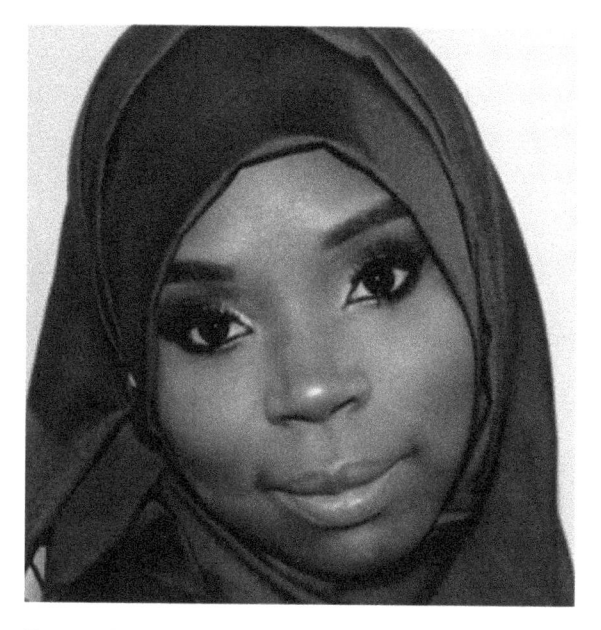

During her teenage years Sophia literally starved herself of love in order to demonstrate the pain she was feeling due to a lack of being able to speak out. But now she's breaking the silence after having realised that the only way to heal was to open up and learn to love; both Allah, but most importantly, herself unconditionally…

I have always believed that I was meant for something more, something deeper, something purer, than what I was subjected to.

Although I had never quite figured out what that something was.

I have now, and I'm living it every day.

I do not know when it actually all began. What I do know is, for as long as I can remember, I felt as though there was no place for me in this world. I now no longer feel that way.

I was unhappy for a long time; I remember thinking and feeling one day at only the tender age of 12 years old that I could not carry on any longer.

I started to starve myself, only living on water and crackers. I used to use a newspaper underneath my plate to hide and tuck away my food, whilst I would watch my family eating, talking and laughing. I only started with dinner, eating only breakfast, then one day I just stopped eating. I did not keep count of how many days or months this went on. I remember occasionally looking in the mirror and not recognising myself and feeling incredibly faint all the time. Then one day I caught a reflection of myself as I lifted my top up. I remember all I could see was bones and then I realised my clothes no longer fitted me.

In my world it was the only thing I could control in the midst of all the changes, the loss I suffered and the pain I felt, and no one was asking questions. Then one day at the dinner table an aunt of mine demanded that I show her what was underneath my newspaper and finally my time was up. It was a series of many things that followed, a way that I could only express that I was hurting, and I needed someone to listen to my pain, my trauma, the trauma that I had suffered at such a young age.

The first time that I thought about suicide was at the age of 16. I had a discussion with myself and I convinced myself that this was the only way forward and nothing else was going to get better. I looked at all the pills that I was beginning to take then suddenly I started crying. I started to think about my dad and how he was cruelly taken away from me out of this world, forever gone and never coming back. How much I missed him, how much I wanted him to be part of my life.

Then I started to call on Allah (God) to give me strength for I felt so weak; at only 16 so much had happened to me and looking at another 16 years of my life felt impossible to endure. I cannot explain in words the events that followed next. I was not really spiritual, but I believed in Allah and I certainly believed in miracles. I felt a wave of comfort envelope me and I sat up, for I do not know how many hours, I just sat and cried until I slept. I believe that Allah saved me that night and I know that He wanted me for better things.

After a few years in therapy, working through my trauma from my childhood, more than sixteen years later, I now feel a lot happier. I have two beautiful children whom I absolutely adore and love myself for allowing them to have me as their mum.

When you are experiencing mental distress, someone is not able to come with a magic wand and wipe away all the past and the pain and unbearable memories it leaves behind. My mental distress was something that I needed to accept and work through with a professional and recognise that, despite the desperation of wanting a quick fix, I needed to value myself and be patient with the healing process. I promise you, just like a broken bone heals, your heart will heal too. I needed to love myself. I needed to understand that I was broken, I was hurt at a young age and it was not my fault. Allah had given me a chance to tell others that there is nothing to be ashamed of, your brokenness is what makes you who you are. It was and it is a part of me and although at times things will be difficult - as life has its ups and downs, it's highs and lows - it does and will get better and the only way when you are down is up.

There were times when I felt ashamed of carrying these wounds as a Muslim, as a practicing Muslim. Praying all my prayers, attending sermons but still feeling hurt, angry and wounded. But I learnt after some time, that Allah loves everyone: broken, wounded, hurt, abused, He *'Al Wadud'* (which is one of Allah's 99 names and means (the most loving)) loves us all in whatever size, form or however emotionally distressed we are. It was the person in the mirror that struggled to love me and accept what we had been through, but without those experiences, the pain, I would not be who I am today.

I was quickly reminded of how fast you can fall back down and not want to get up again, if you do not keep up with the healing process. But I did get up and I did it in style by choosing myself and loving me again, and taking better care of me and Islam is all about self-care and loving yourself!

> *"Tie your camel first, and then put your trust in Allah."*
>
> Hadith Sunan al-Tirmidhī 2517

Ayan expresses her spiritual journey through powerful poetry that speaks to the soul through song

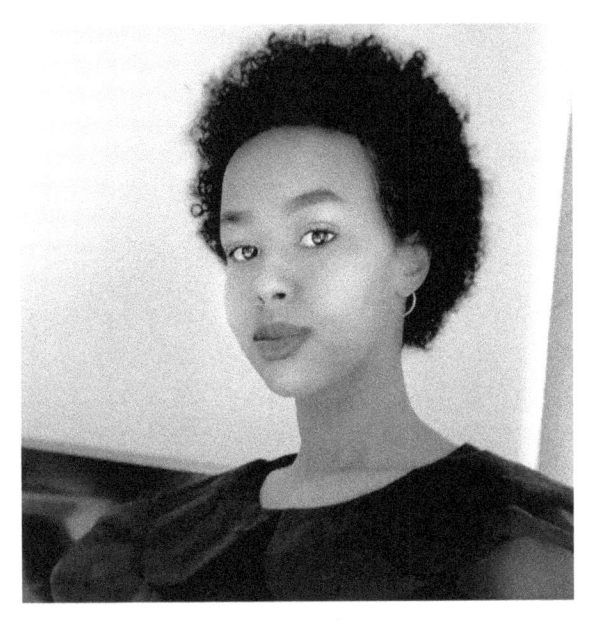

Not all readers may be familiar with the Islamic scriptures and devotion to Allah, and yet the resonance of awakening experience with Ayan's words bridges an uncivilised man-made cultural chasm with an unbreakable bond of love.

When we have …

No name.

No skin colour.

No gender stereotypes.

No man-made culture suppressing us

… if we can surrender enough to listen to our Soul, then humanity can begin to heal the collective traumas that separate us.

Warfare warrior spiritual

Yeah it's a warfare that I am fighting

I am fighting my body to keep standing

Begging my shoulders to stop slouching

Self-image impacting our behavioural patterns and how we see ourselves

Today I allow myself to own the feet it walks on

To feel the ground as I walk towards my dreams

To relax my shoulders and allow my pain to straighten my skeletal

I am tired of getting sucked into dark holes that pull on the strings of my empathy

My emotions aren't open to manipulation from people that fail to see the essence of humanity

I hold no resentment for the spaces that can no longer be in my tomorrow

To be honest it doesn't really matter anymore

I am a spiritual traveller having this human experience, I've been given a vision to pursue whilst I navigate the challenges

It's so intense to hold your pieces together as you face armies that seek to scatter pieces of you.

To be honest I understand all your perspectives but can't respect the way you attack and try to simplify things when it comes to religion and the human condition

You can attempt to identify and place people into boxes

but how about the fact that on some days I have

No name.

No skin colour.

No gender stereotypes.

No man-made culture suppressing me.

How can I be influenced when my soul only seeks to align with the path

Ar-Raheem

I am confident as I elevate to a higher calling

As-Salam

Al-Mumin I am seeking what I failed to find in humans

Al-Muhaymin has seen the journey and now I feel seen as Al-Jabbar restores my faith

I am patient because Ar-Razzaaq saved me from a rat race that had no spiritual purpose

Please leave me in peace as I share dreams with Al-Lateef,

My happiness cannot be thieved when he reminds me every day he is Al-Atheem

How can I get caught up in the whispers when He is Supreme

Speechless

You got me so speechless

Racing to your love

and I swear lately I've been feening like an addict

as I rush to the mat to feel that hit that soothes my soul

and unburdens my problems

Yeah I'm so speechless,

your love has me going senseless

like for real I don't even see things like I use to

and everything I hear now I don't decipher without acknowledging

your presence.

Lord, I am in awe

I'm smelling your nature,

Hypnotised by the geometry of your flowers

and thinking how can the reality of your truth not be taken seriously.

Then I remember me from before,

and how I thought I was the champ, reading and handling life like I had all the answers in a worldly book

I was fuelled by feeding myself worldly qualifications

that I always struggled to swallow because my throat chakra was blocked.

I wasn't aligned

and I kept disconnecting from the connection that had saved me

from every single negative experience.

Yeah you got me speechless

360.

I'm yours and I'm owning it.

Self-expressing freely because I'm at peace in the space of you and I.

Use to live like I was laying on the edges of eggshells anxious of the pain of my steps.

A stranger to my surroundings

Until your light found me, guiding me to the rope

Prayer

My love for God is childlike

Like

I don't want to associate it with anything worldly

But my Lords love is

TOO DIVINE & WISE

For me not to

Translate it into words and language that's c-o-m-p-r-e-h-e-n-s-I-b-l-e

To the human-mind

Because sometimes

some of us struggle to understand.

Just like the way we question the scriptures

Fracturing our spirituality

To gain a fraction of the pleasure we can attain

Right now, I am just focussed on what will remain

After I leave

What will I feel when I am standing before the scale?

How was my character and deeds?

Did I do enough for the deen?

I mean

I am just trying to purify my heart now

Educate myself enough to make sure my unborn children are being raised right

And it hasn't been easy silencing these negative patterns and ways of thinking

But Al-Rahim saved me from the trenches, lifted me from the sorrow I was six feet deep in

Deep this

I was sacrificing my life for people that didn't put a thought into whether I was dead or alive.

How did I expect happiness from a world that didn't even appreciate the blessings before their eyes as they blind themselves to the signs

But Ar-Rahman I am grateful for the mercy

Even though at times I question if I am worthy.

Feeling so undeserving

Constantly practicing protection from the hearsay and whispers Al-Shaytaan uses as a tool to dismantle my emaan into pieces

I owe my becoming to the love you bestowed upon me

I use to swim in the emotions of life, every day felt like I was drowning

Till now, I am still fighting

The difference is I am now floating

In clouds that are so soft to lay in

To break in as my forehead touches the ground in submission

Thank you

For the way you wipe my tears as I plead to you for guidance to build this home so it transcends beyond the skies and waits for me in heaven

My prayer is the reason I can even function as a human

My scriptures taught me things that set my scientific brain on a trajectory that allowed me to analyse everything beyond our visual reality

Indulging in a greatness that's deadening old skin cells and creating new neurons that place me at the centre of my soul

Still struggling but my thirst for knowledge and your love has me falling in love with parts of me I didn't even know existed.

I know I may fall off but I also know aouthu billahi minal shaytaanal rajeem

Grateful for the way you redeemed my hope

I have faith you'll always remind me of the strength that'll keep me on the path

Imran's emotional struggles date back a thousand years, and yet his voice is a current leading light for the Muslim male community

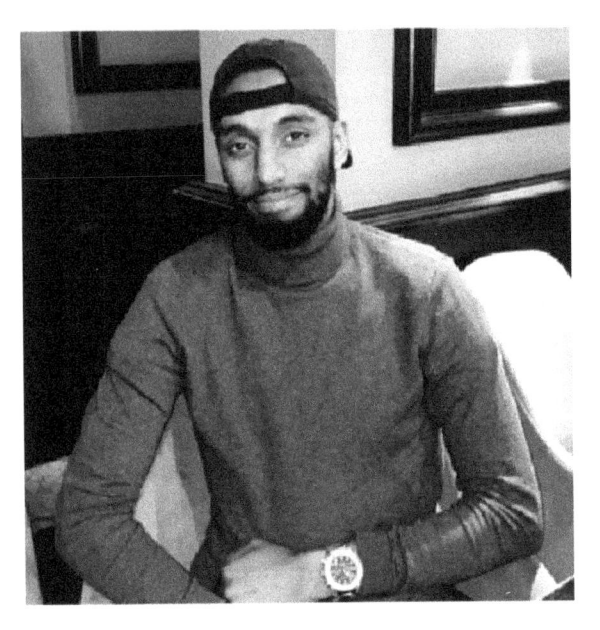

Imran, particularly knows how men in some Muslim communities are expected to provide and 'be strong' for their families and culture. And yet he also knows from the bottom of his heart and soul that "It is actually the strong who admit defeat, who admit when they are in pain"

Imran is a leading voice for his ancestors and his community, and we are so proud of him for speaking out about his struggles. Here is HIStory...

My Story

The lockdown was a challenging time for me and my family. I had been working in a job that I was happy with, I had a supportive team, and even some of them had become my friends. But I was not in the job I studied for, and it was not my field. This lay heavy on my shoulders, and so I kept applying for other jobs - I almost got used to receiving the endless rejection letters.

After two years of constant applications and failed interviews, one day I received an email informing me that I was successful. I went through 3 stages: an online test, a practical exercise, and a zoom Q&A interview. I had successfully passed all 3 stages and was offered the job. It was my dream come true, the duaa (prayer) that I had been making for two years, had finally been accepted by Allah (God). This was the best news I had received since leaving university. I gave in my notice at work, my family, friends and everyone were incredibly happy for me. The job offer was with a big company, it came with a big pay package and staff benefits that could help me and my family get far in life. My previous workplace threw me a massive farewell party and the messages of congratulations were overwhelmingly supportive.

The first few days of my new workplace were challenging. I was given my first task with a deadline. I spent hours on the task, but I did not understand what I was supposed to do. My position was a junior member of staff in the company and during my interview I was reassured that I would be eased into my position. This task did not feel junior at all. After spending hours on end trying to complete the task, I contacted a friend who was in a similar role. He took his time out from his job to help me and even he was surprised at the lack of support I was given and the task that I was instructed to complete. Unfortunately, he could not always give me a hand as he had his own job to get on with.

I finally plucked up the courage and I asked my manager and the person who appointed me to support me. I contacted my manager as the role was online, but he informed me that he was too busy. When I finally got a chance, he gave me about 15 minutes of his time then he would need to go again. His explanations about the task were brief, rushed and caused me further confusion.

Within a week, I started to experience what is known as 'imposter syndrome'. This is when a person who is fully qualified for a position feels like they are unqualified and does not deserve to be there. This started affecting my mental health and I became frustrated with myself and stress started to impact on my sleep and eating. I spent early mornings, late evenings and weekends just trying to work out my task. I began to feel that I could not continue with this role; the pressure was mounting but I promised myself I would not give up and I would keep going until I succeeded.

After two and a half weeks my manager organised a meeting with me. It was named a progress meeting. I was preparing myself to inform the company of the struggles I was having. My meeting lasted what felt like a few minutes. I was told that I was not up to the expectations they needed, it was not working out for them, so they had to release me and let me go. I was so shocked that the only thing that I could say was "okay, okay" and that was it. I had lost my dream job in a few minutes. I felt a sigh of relief, then feelings of shame and anger started pouring in. I had no strength to fight the decision, I was frozen, confused, hurt. I sat numbly at my work desk at home and everything around me was blurred. How was I going to tell my family? I still had "congratulations on your new job" messages from my previous workplace, which every time I read felt like a bullet of failure hitting me; a voice inside of me said "Imran, you're an embarrassment". I felt so worthless, and I kept calling myself "stupid".

For three weeks, I woke up and sat at my work desk. I could not bring myself to tell anyone what had happened, not even my close friends. No one knew that I woke up every morning and got ready for a job that I had lost. The hours I spent pretending to still have a job were painful; feelings of unworthiness, not being good enough and like I had lost everything. I started to question Allah (God), why would he give me something and just take it away? Maybe this was what I deserved, maybe this was it. One of the main struggles I felt was that my prayers were not going anywhere.

Then one day I lost the will to pretend anymore. I just did not get up for work that day. My family were concerned and questioned me, and I finally told them the bad news that I had lost my job. I felt like I'd let myself, my family, and my friends down. I started becoming anxious when I saw job adverts in my field, and I felt that I would never ever be able to apply again.

My depression hit a very low point during those months. I was jobless and struggling to find work as it was during the peak of the Covid-19 pandemic. I hit rock bottom. I could not provide for myself, nor my family. "I have failed in my role as a man", is what I kept telling myself.

I always painted a picture of happiness and smiles to everyone around me but inside I was filled with sadness and pain. I did not want to show or share how I felt because I felt that, as a man, I should be 'tough' and be able to get through this. I often found writing was a means to relieve myself of any of my problems. This was one of the many poems that I had written during those times:

> *Take a look and see life through my eyes,*
> *Maybe you will understand the way that I feel inside,*
> *Maybe you will realise that deep down I'm broken,*
> *and the blood flowing through me is now frozen,*
> *became accustomed to the pain and disappointment,*
> *happiness is now a language that's not spoken,*
> *with every joy comes a rain full of problems,*
> *now I realise why my smile is just a wash away...*

Looking back now with hindsight I feel like my manager set me up to fail. After finally speaking to a few of my friends they highlighted the fact that I had received no induction, I did not shadow anyone, and the one person appointed to support me was always unavailable. I had been expected to hit the ground running. That feeling of relief that I had first felt when I lost my job had been my intuition, telling me that probably it was not the right place for me to work. Sometimes I question myself why I did not call the meeting myself and be confident enough to say, "you are not supporting me" that actually, although it was my dream job it was not working out for me either.

Sometimes we put so much emphasis on where we should be. Where we should be going. We forget to live in the present...

I did learn some lessons, although some were painful, I also learnt a lot about myself. It is so difficult for men to always look strong and have everything under control. It is actually the strong who admit defeat, who admit when they are in pain. Defeat is not failure; it is to surrender and accept that the situation is not suited to you. It is allowing ourselves to pause and reflect. No job, no amount of money, is ever worth your mental health.

One of Allah's names is *'Ar Razzaq'*- which means: The Provider, The Sustainer, The Bestower of Sustenance. Indeed, He Ar-Razaaq did grant me another job where I was able to provide for my family. Though not my dream job yet, I believe when the time is right that job will come with the right support.

Who am I?

Three powerful words that unlock a story, filled with a thousand chapters, dated back to a time when man still lit fire with sticks.

A question that forces the past to merge with the present. That drags the roots from every tree welded deep within the ground.

That traces my D.N.A, in the soil, well beyond a million miles: who am I?

I... couldn't answer that alone, not without the voices of my ancestors echoing over me.

I am a master puzzle piece, pieced together from every nation and tribe, herb and spice.

But what you see is only a form of clay, like when a caterpillar breaks open to become a butterfly.

So, believe me when I tell you, there is more to me on the inside.

Who am I? ... I need to look beyond the reflection of every eyeball that stares at me.

Beyond the racial slurs and hatred words that try to portray me, that try to tell me who I am, without even asking me.

Well, it's a good thing they don't.

Because when they finally do.

I'll have to reply with a thousand chapters, dated back to a time when man still lit fire with sticks.

Sara knows that the divine path she is walking as a Muslim Psychologist is no coincidence

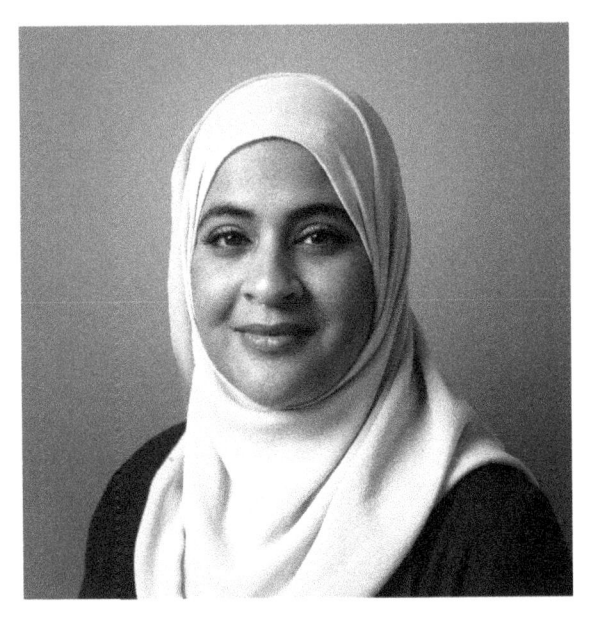

Dr Sara is no stranger to mental health; she grew up around Psychiatric Hospitals and 'returned home' to learn that this may not be providing the safest of spaces to her fellow Muslims, or in fact, anyone struggling with mental distress. Here Sara bravely shares her journey within the NHS system - its downfalls - and her wisdom about how we might better serve our fellow humans to honour suffering and beliefs as they need to be honoured...

I remember being 11 years old and vowing that I would never work in a hospital.

Having now spent nearly 20 years working in and out of hospitals I look back and smile at the steely determination of that 11-year-old and wonder about fate and destiny and God's plan.

My parents both migrated to this country and spent their entire working lives as nurses in NHS Mental Health Services. When I was born in the early 1980s, we were living in nurses' accommodation, on the grounds of a big old Victorian 'Psychiatric Institution'. These institutions were often purposefully built in the countryside away from main society (as they felt the 'patients' should be kept away) but for us it meant living in nice houses in affluent leafy areas. My parents' whole lives revolved around this place; their work, their social networks, friends, support, community, everyone was in some-way connected to the hospital. I remember Christmas parties and ward events in which, as children, we were occasionally allowed to attend. I was greatly intrigued by this weird and wonderful workplace. It didn't scare me the way it probably would most children, I always felt honoured to be there, with a strange mix of sadness and excitement and an overwhelming sense that these people, for some reason, really needed to be cared for.

After a brief stint as a chambermaid and then at Sainsbury's, by the age of 17 I was working as a Care Assistant in a nursing home that my dad helped to manage for adults with severe mental health issues, and have remained in the field ever since. I remember in one of the very first places I worked, I cared for an elderly man who recognised my surname. It transpired that he had been the manager of a 'psychiatric ward' that my dad had worked in the late 1970s. It was an odd moment for us both, it felt like he had come full circle in the strange way that often happens in life and for me it felt like a validation that I was supposed to be there. I have that same sense now when I think about my career, that in some strange way, I have come back home.

In the years following, I got my degree in Psychology (still not wanting to work in hospitals) and continued working part time in Learning Disability and Mental Health facilities to earn money. I began to understand this world of mental distress a little better, not only by the people I was working with, but by becoming increasingly aware of close family members experiencing mental distress. I became aware of the cultural stigma around mental health and when my relative became so unwell that he needed support from outside services, I was faced with a barrier of silence and inaction from the family. I was the only one willing to acknowledge this situation, make difficult decisions, have difficult conversations, and face difficult truths. Looking back at this event I can hardly believe it happened. I attended a conference last year about being a 'Stranger in a City' in which it explored the research findings that if you migrate to an area in which you become a minority it is significantly more likely that you will experience serious mental distress. This was indeed what had happened to my relative, along with drug use (to manage the difficult feelings he was experiencing), complicated and difficult family relationships and history, lack of work/study, and social isolation, which all created a traumatic concoction resulting in him experiencing visions and voices of a scary nature. These 'symptoms' led to him being sectioned under the Mental Health Act and having a long hospital stay, after which, he went back home to his country of origin. I am grateful to say that he has since reconnected with God and found his spirituality, given up the drug use and found some purpose and meaning to his life and is in a much better place now.

My journey with God started from a very young age. I always felt aware that the world we see in front of us isn't all that is there. Despite not coming from a religious family, I went to Christian schools and so God was always a positive quiet presence in the background of my home and school life. I taught myself how to pray the Muslim prayers mainly in an attempt to pass my GCSEs and hoped that if I prayed to Him properly, He would grant me that. My best friend and I were also always slightly intrigued (albeit very scared) of 'other worldly' things and would spend many hours wondering what else was out there. Looking back now I would say that I have always been 'sensitive' to other things that may be around, and from my Muslim faith I would interpret those things now as being Angels and Jinn, but back then I just had a sense that we weren't alone. These early feelings solidified my belief in God, but the full connection lay slightly dormant until my late 20s when it awoke with the jolt of a few difficult years of getting divorced, being diagnosed with Crohn's disease, and applying for Psychology Doctoral training.

Having come from a very white middle class area in the leafy suburbs of Surrey to working in some of the poorest parts of East London, I'd had a massive culture shock. As a young naïve Assistant Psychologist, I met a Clinical Psychologist who wore the full length very loose black dress (abaya) and black head scarf (hijab). I had never met anyone like her before. She was my senior; confident, stern, held her own in very intimidating 'psychology meetings' and I didn't know what to make of her. Although I was slightly scared of her I sensed that she saw more in me and made it her job to help me along my journey. I owe it to that sister (may Allah reward her) for gently pushing me onto the 'formal start' of my Islamic journey, she bought me my first hijab and I have not looked back since. Not long after this I got accepted onto the Psychology Doctorate course, and so my journey with Islam and God has always run alongside my journey of becoming a Psychologist, the two are very much interwoven.

As I was finishing my Doctorate, I decided to take a post as a Muslim Chaplain in the Mental Health Trust I was working in to begin to bring together my skills as a Psychologist with my faith. This is some of the most rewarding work I have ever done, but it was also one of the most difficult jobs I have ever had (and I've worked in some very challenging places!). Although I was employed by the NHS as a Spiritual Care Advisor/Chaplain, services generally were not really interested in meeting the religious and spiritual needs of patients in the most important sense and I saw many Muslim patients in great distress emotionally, psychologically, and spiritually. I was there for 5 years and during that time I received large numbers of referrals regarding issues around Jinn, Evil Eye and Black Magic. By this time, I had been working in Mental Health Services for nearly 15 years and what was becoming very apparent to me was that the system we have currently does not work for the majority of people who use it. In fact, most people with severe difficulties stay in the system for most of their lives, often becoming more unwell from the side effects of the strong medication. I was shocked to find out that there are a lot of research papers and national reports that spell this out in black and white and say that the system is unsustainable and needs to change. It devastates me that even years after many of these reports were published I can see no real change in the culture of how we treat people in distress, and in some situations it is now worse. I was even more devastated to find out that there is also a lot of research to back up another distressing thing I was witnessing daily; that the system is even less likely to work for you (and in many cases abuse and neglect you disproportionately more) if you are from a black or 'ethnic minority' background. I had become traumatised by years of watching patients in mental distress be treated worse than animals. People were treated like they were a problem, like what was happening to them was their fault, like they were not human anymore, they were neglected in their hours of need, or worse they would be medicated to silence their distress. The knowledge that this was intensified if you happened to look like me or my family, is heartbreaking.

Whilst the medication can sometimes help with some of the symptoms, it certainly is not the cure. Every part of my being told me that this was not purely some physical disease, but that these people had gone through - or were still going through - something terrible in their lives and for whatever reason had not recovered. I knew in my heart that the healing would come through listening to and understanding their distress. I also learned that not only was the mental health system and the way that we treat (all) people with mental distress traumatising to me, but that after 20 years I was also traumatised by the institutional racism that affects both the patients and staff every-single-day.

As my faith in the mental health system began to rapidly decrease, and my knowledge of more psychological and spiritual aspects of mental health increased, and at a time when I thought I was not going to be able to continue working in the NHS mental health system as it is, I was guided to a model called Open Dialogue. In the 1980s Finland had some of the highest rates of people who were experiencing severe mental distress; seeing and hearing things that others couldn't and having unusual thoughts and beliefs, that they decided to try something different to the predominant western model and eventually 'Open Dialogue' evolved over the following years. Whilst I cannot fully explain the model here, I hope to express some of its essence; this model is based on the notion that whatever someone is expressing when they are in severe mental distress – even if we can't understand them – *is meaningful*. That the things they see and hear, the strange and unusual ideas and beliefs they have, are connected in some way to a distress or trauma in their lives that they haven't been able to process and move on from – essentially they have remained stuck in their distress. This model works with the person and their whole family/network, it's a model based on equality as humans (removing the clinician as expert dynamic), it seeks to provide help as soon as possible and for as long as the patient and their family need it. The principles are best described in non-technical terms as compassion, mercy, love and kindness – hearing and holding everyone's different views and distress and pain and providing a space for families to process life's difficulties, to understand them and begin to heal. My heart knew instantly that this is the way we should be working with anyone in mental distress, it reminds me of the verse that Muslims repeat often many times a day:

"Bismillah-hir-Rahmaan-nir-Raheem"

"God is the Most Merciful, the Most Kind, the Most Compassionate"

Sure enough, over the last 30 years the hospital in Finland (Western Lapland) has gone from 4 wards down to 1; it has some of the best results worldwide for working with the diagnosis psychiatry calls 'psychosis' and has proven that with a model that treats the person (even the most severe) as being in a meaningful state of distress, people who have been unwell for many years have made a full recovery, without the need for life long medication.

Whilst working with Muslim communities in mental health services I slowly began to make connections with all the things I had learnt in the last 20 years. As a Muslim I believe that every human is made up of a physical body, a life force (Ruh), a spiritual heart (the 'Qalb' our control centre that houses our thoughts, emotions, intentions, intelligence, reasoning and direct connection to God- Fitrah) and a soul (Nafs – the part that drives the other parts). I believe that part of the test of this life is to learn to control our soul (and therefore whole self) and work on developing it to be the best version of itself as it has equal potential for good and bad. I also believe that we have an enemy called Satan whose sole purpose is to mislead us and make us fall. As a psychologist I believe that every human (and all their parts mentioned above) is impacted greatly by the events that happen to them, how they experience life, relationships, love, trauma, God, and that all experiences form lasting effects on the heart, body and soul. If those life experiences combine in a negative way, for example a child is born with a very nervous nature, they are then abused by a person in a position of authority- perhaps a family member – and as they grow older this causes them to disconnect from God and become angry at why God let this happen, Satan continues to whisper negative thoughts about them lowering their already beaten sense of self-worth. And then, when one day they lose their job after many of life's struggles, or get divorced, or fail exams, or face a close bereavement, what do you think would happen? I think life would become very hard, thoughts would become very dark, and that connection to God becomes clouded – even for people who are praying 5 times a day.

There are themes to the tests in life that God tells us about in the Quran, He will test us with fear, and loss, and death, and poverty, and Satan tells us how he will make it all far worse. A slow build spanning years, an unfortunate combination, and a final straw can make a person who appears on the outside as a 'good decent Muslim from a good family' suddenly crack and dismantle from the inside until they are unrecognisable and incomprehensible. If you add to that our beliefs in black magic and evil eye, jealousy and envy, you have the perfect recipe for extreme mental distress.

By now you must be thinking why on earth would God put us through all of this? What is the point? The point is that it is one of the main purposes of this life to go through pain and distress in order to purify our hearts and souls and connect to God in the purest way, fully subservient and humble. This is known as the 'greater jihaad' or the 'great inner struggle of the self'. To pull ourselves back to God despite the things that happen to us. Every pain is to bring us closer to Him. Many of my clients have told me that in their darkest days of hearing voices and seeing things this was also when they were the most aware of God's existence, they could feel the other world and often became very religious in those moments.

But I believe there is also another reason for all this distress, that these tests are for us as an Ummah (Muslim Community) too, and they are here to help us elevate as an Ummah. If our Ummah could learn to treat our brothers and sisters who have severe mental distress with compassion, mercy, love and kindness, it will surely be one of the deeds that raises our status as an Ummah, because in order to do this *we all* have to change, *we all* have to learn the true acts of compassion and mercy and let go of anger, resentment, pain and power.

Last year my aunt (in another country), who had lived most of her 50 years in a psychiatric hospital, died. The pain I felt upon her death pierces my heart every time I think of her. I won't list her traumas here, but there were many. There were difficult family relationships, there was a lack of understanding and an unwillingness from the family to see that they would need to change their ways to heal this, maybe even some black magic thrown in, and suddenly there she was – a teenager seeing things, hearing things, screaming, crying, hysterical and angry. But also, funny and bright and beautiful, she could speak 3 languages despite having to leave school because of the 'illness'. She became the 'ill one' for decades until finally at age 50 she gave up on life and slowly just stopped living, and God took her soul. The pain for me is on many levels. I have spent my career caring for people like her but could do nothing for her. I learnt a model of treatment that had the potential to heal her but I couldn't offer her that. I can see all the family issues but am too distant to help. Her once beautiful face taken away by the years of torment and strong drugs will always haunt me, but it also pushes me to keep going.

It is no coincidence that both my parents were mental health nurses and that I was born on the grounds of an old psychiatric hospital, it is no coincidence I have many significant family experiences of severe mental distress, it is no coincidence that I found Open Dialogue in this big wide world, and it is no coincidence that I am sitting here writing this story. I feel connected to my fate and put my trust in God. He has brought me here to this point and will continue to guide me if I ask and listen.

I now march side by side with a growing group of people from all walks of life, all faiths, all colours, all races, standing together fighting to change the western model of mental health care. To remove it from the medical world of diagnosis and drugs and individualistic treatments, to a more holistic compassionate approach which values psychological, spiritual, social, relational, natural approaches to healing alongside medication and 1-1 treatments (when needed and wanted). An approach which offers space, time, community, and healing. An approach that understands that it's not just chemical imbalances, or only thoughts and feelings, that have been affected but that it is also a person's connection to God. I believe as a Muslim Psychologist and Compassionate Mental Health Activist that people can lose their way in life's traumas big and small, and they need help from us to find their way back; that it takes a community and many different approaches to do that. As an Ummah we have to be prepared to hear the horror stories and change our ways, to not judge and condemn, to not ignore or deny, to not mock and ridicule, because none of us (or our families) are immune to experiencing mental distress in any way, but to listen and support, to be just and caring, to give time and understanding, and because;

"Whosoever relieves from a believer some grief pertaining to this world, Allah will relieve from him some grief pertaining to the Hereafter".
Hadith Muslim 1508 Book 16
The Comprehensive Book Sahih Muslim.

Find out more about Sara's work here:
www.Dr-Sara.com

Waheedah has transformed the pain of her loss into a philosophical reflection on the journey of life

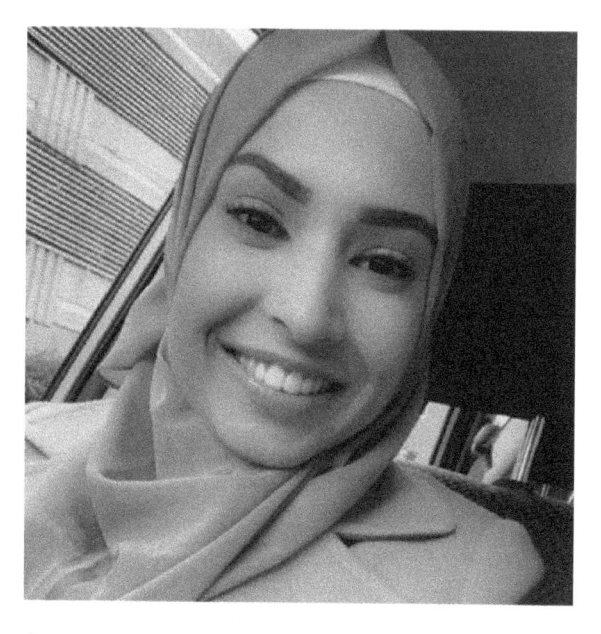

Sometimes it can be the most devastating circumstances that create the deepest bonds. Waheedah's experience of losing one of her most loved family members twice almost broke her, but she's back on the train of life and enjoying witnessing the growing bonds between her own daughter and father. Here Waheedah shares her story of love and loss ...

My Sister

My sister was my best friend and although we were four boys and two girls, the eldest three were like a triangle support for the siblings. We played, fought, argued, and loved each other tremendously. My father and mother brought us up to love, value and respect one another. We knew the importance of family and did everything together.

On December 2007 my sister got married and moved to England from Germany where we all lived. I was 12 years old and I did not realise what was happening. Not only because everything happened so fast, but also because I had an important soccer game on that day. I remember it like it was yesterday. The wedding was in my aunt's beautiful garden, everyone was saying goodbye. We hugged, my sister entered the car and shut the door. As soon as we started waving, she began to cry. We also started crying. I still remember her driving away. At night I realised that she had gone for good when I noticed her side of the bedroom we shared was empty. Her cupboard was also empty, I felt her absence. She was already missing.

The first years after she left, we talked every day for hours. I told her about my school, I shared with her my fears, my hopes and my dreams; most importantly, I always asked her opinion about everything. She told me a little less about married life but seldom allowed me to do the talking.

When I heard my sister was pregnant it was so exciting, our first nephew or niece, my parents' first grandchild. I kept imagining how much I would spoil them. As she got closer to her labour, my mum, brother and I booked a ticket from Germany to be with her in England. We packed baby clothes and everything we thought she was going to need; it was the first time I was going to see her since she had left. We got to the airport but were blocked from travelling because my mum did not have a visa. My dream had burst. I started crying. We came home, unpacked and told her the bad news. It was a difficult and sad conversation. She was upset. She felt lonely. She continued to miss our company.

Then in summer 2012 my elder brother and I were finally able to visit her. This was the first time I realised and accepted that she was married now with a new life, her own family. Although everything seemed to be going well when we visited my sister, I noticed that something was not right. She had lost a lot of weight. She'd started telling me about the diets she was trying and the slimming tablets she was taking. My heart sank and it hit me that she was going through an eating disorder. Flying back home, I felt so helpless even though I'd spent the days I had left with her telling her that she was perfect, that she did not need to lose any weight, she was convinced that she was overweight.

Two summers later, we were back in England to visit my sister as she had given birth to my beautiful niece. My niece was about 6 days old, my sister came home from the hospital and I noticed she had an obvious lump on her back. My sister was holding a letter in her hand and tears were rolling down her face. When I asked her what was wrong, she told me the lump on her back was cancer. The word cancer rang in my ears, I couldn't believe it. When I called my mum and dad to tell them the news it was surreal, as if I were watching someone else's life. I told my sister that it was okay, she would be fine, that so many people had healed from cancer and I honestly believed this. I kept telling myself it was not as if her cancer had spread, we could see the lump and all the surgeons had to do was to remove it. Everything sounded easy and manageable. It sounded like a story with a happy ending.

The following months were like a storm had hit my family and pulled us apart with pain and sorrow. We kept going backwards and forwards with misinformation on my sister's condition. Then, when she came to stay with us again, I had my sister back for a few days. When she was back in England, after her first operation, she became incredibly sick, and we stopped hearing from her.

Whilst in Germany, one of my mum's sisters called one day as she recalled a chilling dream, and because of my sister's condition we did not want to take any chances. We packed our bags and headed back to England where my sister was. We did not even know where my sister lived. We received some information from a relative and we frantically started knocking on doors and I listened for familiar sounds. I heard a voice moaning and I knew it was my sister. It sounded like she wanted to cry but at the same time was trying to be strong. It sounded like she wanted to scream but couldn't, it sounded like she was suffering.

When we entered the room, it was exactly how my aunt had described in her dream. It was obvious she had been through difficult chemotherapy treatment. My sister looked at us and thought she was dreaming. She thought that it was the morphine that had made her hallucinate seeing us there. My mum squeezed her hand gently and told her she was not dreaming. We were speechless and shocked.

I did not recognize my sister, I felt like my family had failed and I had failed as a sister. My father suffered a lumbago, and he was diagnosed with internal bleeding. Finding my sister in that state broke my heart and for the first time since her cancer diagnosis, I realised she was going to die. I started questioning Allah. Why are we being tested like this? Why us? Why everything in one go? Why do you want to take my only sister away from me?

'Do the people think that they will be left to say, "We believe" and they will not be tried? But We have certainly tried those before them, and Allah will surely make evident those who are truthful, and He will surely make evident those who are false.'
Qur'an Surah Al-'Ankabut, 29: 2-3

After questioning everything I started seeing the whole situation from a different perspective. Allah tests us to purify us and wash away our sins. These tests are given to us to strengthen our Iman (faith). And most importantly: Allah tests a person He loves. I stopped thinking "why us?" and instead thought "***Ya Rahman***. The one who is most kind, loving and merciful. Allhamdullah, another test."

The nurse who came to administer the morphine told us they were just giving her palliative care. Her wounds were seeping and refusing to heal from a recent surgery. Her only wish that day was to shop for Eid clothes for her children. My brother carried her in a wheelchair and we took her shopping. Even when we were choosing clothes, she would fall asleep for a few minutes due to the morphine then wake up begging us to carry on. I admired the strength she carried, and I was ashamed for feeling so broken for her.

I wish I had told her how strong I thought she was, and how I admired her bravery that even when she cried, I knew she was in pain, but she would not want me to see her hurting. Cancer changes the body but not the soul. The soul is still the person you know and love.

On the journey back home, I could not take the image of my sister from my mind. Her last words to me were how much she loved me. I told my mum I could not go back and that she should stay with my sister and I would take care of my younger brothers and our family home.

The following days were so clear, each day weighed heavily on my shoulders, I was receiving one piece of bad news after another. My world had stopped, my family was in pieces. I found eating difficult, it was as if all the joys and all the laughter we shared had been sucked out of us. Her heart was still beating but it felt like she was gone; she could not really talk anymore, she couldn't eat anymore. Her eyes were closed. We were all in this dark tunnel just waiting for the inevitable. As I took care of my younger brothers whilst my mum, dad, and eldest brother stayed in England with my sister, we felt that our world was shattering.

On Saturday the 16th of August 2014 I could not eat, my heart and mind were with my sister. The following day I remember receiving the text message a few minutes before 9 am, that my beautiful sister had departed from this world.

I miss you
Nothing hurts like not seeing you
And no one understands what we went through
It was short. It was sweet. You died.

It feels like it was just recently,
Staying up all night telling each other stories secretly.
I cannot describe how much I miss your company.

The biggest shock in my life was hearing that you have cancer,
A sickness that kills and tortures,
A sickness that not everyone defeats.

Seeing you suffering, crying, and fighting,
Seeing you trying, praying, and hoping,
Seeing the sickness killing you slowly,
Not seeing the real Aneesah - was killing me inside.

Sitting helplessly next to you,
Telling stories that we made,
Knowing that any breath could be your last one,
Hoping that the moment would never end.

It was time to leave,
Telling each other goodbye,
It didn't feel like I would see you again,
Looking at you, while your eyes were closing and tears falling off my eyes. "I love you Waheedah.", were your last words to me.

I miss you
Nothing hurts like not seeing you
And no one understands what we went through
It was short. It was sweet. You died.

May You Rest In Peace my sister. 17.08.2014

I named my daughter Aneesah Liya…

Liya meaning - Most beautiful form of patience (Arabic) - lioness (Latin) as strong as Aneesah also meaning the highest level of sabr (patience).

I told our neighbors the news and so many guests came to visit. At first, I could not cry. Then the imam (spiritual leader) who had conducted my sister's wedding came into the house limping due to a recent surgery, he was crying silently. That is when it dawned on me that my sister had passed on. I began to cry and everyone in the house was weeping, it was truly a sorrowful day. I did not leave my room for three or four hours. I stayed in the dark. I was broken and I desperately missed her so much.

My parents came back the following morning after my sister's burial, the whole neighborhood gathered to give their condolences. I could not take my eyes off my father, my father was a tall strong man, but that day I could see that both my parents were enveloped by grief. For my parents, their eldest daughter dying from cancer at the tender age of only 27 years old was devastating. They say grief comes in stages, but I believe it is different for everyone. For me, it was when I was at the supermarket and saw sisters together. When my friends talked about their sisters my loss was heightened in volumes. I'd lost my best friend, my elder sister, and the light of our life. She was sweet, gentle, and had a heart of gold. It's the little things I think we take for granted like that extra hug or just staying a little longer on the phone. My grief hit me harder when I got married and I was pregnant with my first daughter. Grief grips you by surprise, it can be something that she found funny, or her favourite food, or just childhood memories that overwhelm our family festive days.

My dad bought a Bonsai tree - which would be the same age as Aneesah, he said it was a symbol of her. He takes care of the tree, with the right balance, not too much water or too little, he keeps this tree in his room with a picture of Aneesah, even when he is sick, he must look after the Bonsai tree, my father would sit for hours just staring at the tree.

When I named my daughter Aneesah, I also wanted a name that could describe how Aneesah was, for me I wanted to hear my sister and then my daughter. My father held my daughter and he saw her, and he suddenly began to cry then he said, "I remember this is how I held Aneesah years ago and now she is just gone." I can see that my father loves Aneesah so much, he is always telling her about her aunty Aneesah and showing her pictures which is so lovely. Even though my daughter has not replaced my sister, she has helped me put back a piece of the missing puzzle, not completely, but she is a beautiful addition to my family.

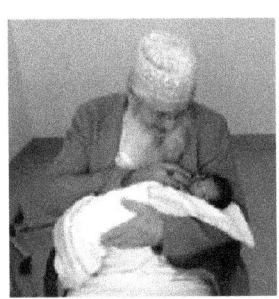

Even though we miss her, I see this as a journey.

This life is just a journey, we are all just passing through, it is like being on the train, whenever anyone is at the train station, we do not know who is leaving, it happens when it is your time. I guess

my sister left because she was already at the door...
Some people leave who are younger, older, sick or healthy ...

This painful experience has brought us together as a family.

> *"And whoever relies upon Allah -*
> *then He is sufficient for him".*
> Qur'an Surah At-Talāq, 65:3

Alina is Proud that her struggles have given her the strength to develop hope and belief in herself

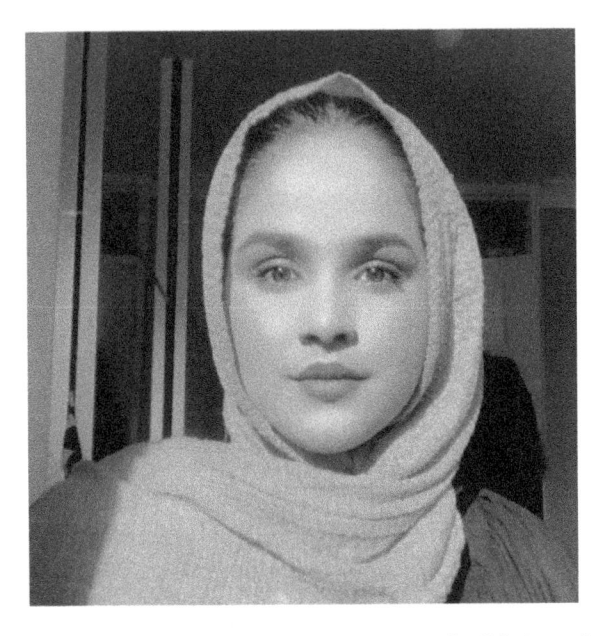

At only 19, Alina has already experienced a lifetime of chronic illness, but rather than let it destroy her spirit, she is proud to be focusing on her dreams and accepting of any natural emotions that surface along the way... We are proud of you too Alina!

The Girl with a Story

Hello, my name's Alina and my story begins on the 16th July 2017. It's the day my entire life changed. It's the day my upper limb gave up on me. It's the day I could no longer fend for myself, take care of myself, or do anything for myself. From that very day on, I slowly lost the ability to fully function all of my limbs like I used to be able to. From that very day on, life had completely and utterly changed for me. I was eventually diagnosed with a lifelong, auto-immune chronic nerve pain illness - Complex Regional Pain Syndrome. I never knew pain could be so debilitating, so excruciating. My entire life had changed in under 24 hours.

As you can imagine, being left bed-bound, unable to fend for myself, unable to do anything for myself, had a horrible negative effect on my mental health. There was (and still is) no cure for my illness - I was simply a 16-year-old who spent most of her time in hospital or in bed, crying her eyes out. I tried to fight through the pain, but I was not getting anywhere. I felt suffocated. I was living a life I did not want to live. I struggled to cope with what life was throwing at me. I developed anxiety and experienced months of sadness. I could not see the light at the end of the tunnel. I did not want to be alive with all this pain anymore.

Prior to developing my illness, I had always been a happy, hard-working person. I always wanted to strive to be the best at whatever it was I was doing – I was a little perfectionist. I loved studying and wanted to go to university one day to pursue my dreams. I was due to start sixth form in September 2017 and I was determined to get there - I just didn't know how. With the amazing support of my parents and teachers, I managed to get myself into sixth form on most days. There were days where I could not physically make it to school. There were days where I physically could not make it to my lessons. I always tried my best and I am so grateful for the teachers who supported me. However, school had not always been positive for me. As I physically look completely fine, many of my peers did not believe I was battling a chronic illness. I heard constant remarks about myself from others. I had constant remarks being made about how I was 'faking' my illness, how I was 'pretending for attention'. As you can imagine this slowly was, both mentally and physically, destroying me. It took me a very long time before I was able to stand up for myself. There came a day where I had simply had enough of all the hurtful remarks, of physically being pushed around, of mentally being hurt by these people. I finally stood my ground and told them to leave me alone, to let me be. It was the most frightening thing I had ever done but deep down I knew it was the only way I could get my point across, the only way I'd be able to make school life better for myself.

All of these events had made my anxiety and sadness worse. I was beginning to struggle even more with learning to cope with the pain and over the last few years, I was diagnosed with more conditions and was experiencing more symptoms. I am now 20 years old and suffer from Complex Regional Pain Syndrome, Fibromyalgia, Chronic Widespread Pain, IBS symptoms, Anxiety and I am also being investigated for POTS, a tachycardia syndrome. I have come a very long way with dealing with my debilitating pains and symptoms. I have taught myself how to use my limbs again, how to walk again. It has been the most difficult few years of my life, but I am so grateful for it all. Islam has played a huge part in helping me learn how to cope. I began to see my illnesses as a blessing rather than a curse. Praying helps me to get through my days. Of course, to this day, there are still times where I am so mentally and physically drained from trying to manage everything, from trying to fight through the pain, from trying to keep going, but I try my very best. During these times, I try to give myself time and space to 'heal', to cope with what I am going through.

If there is one thing that my chronic illness and mental health struggles have taught me, it is the fact that everyone has something they are going through behind closed doors. Kindness is something that does not cost a penny yet many still choose to not use it. By going through what I have and am still going through, I have become a much more understanding person. Life isn't always easy but if there's one thing that I know and strongly believe in, it's that no soul is put through more than they can handle. This life is a test and those who have the hardest tests in this life have rewards waiting for them on the other end that are beyond what you can even imagine. I always try my best to remember this and most of the time it gets me through my days. However, there are still days where, no matter how positive I try to be, I cannot help but break down, I cannot help but cry and that's okay! It is unhealthy for someone to have no 'bad' days, it is unhealthy for someone to remain positive 24/7. You have to let yourself let out all your emotions. Having a 'bad day' does not make you weak, it simply shows you how incredibly strong you really are.

During my first year and a half of diagnosis, I struggled so very much to cope with life, school, my education, etc. As I mentioned earlier, I did not see the light at the end of the tunnel, I did not have much hope for my future. However, I did not give up. I kept pushing through, every single day, and I still do. I have now just finished my sixth form studies and am due to start university in a few months to pursue my dreams Insha'Allah.

I never ever thought I'd be where I am now. I never ever imagined myself to have gotten this far. Hope and belief in yourself is something that is so very important. Never give up! You can handle whatever it is you are going through, I promise you that. Be kind to yourself, look after yourself, put yourself first – these are things I am still working on, but I know they are very important.

I have an Instagram page set up @thegirlwithastory to raise awareness of chronic illness and to be part of a support network if anyone needs it.

> *"Al-Jabbar - The Powerful Restorer"*
> Name and attribute of God (Allah)

Faduma emerges through depression, hearing voices, disordered eating and embracing a son with unique needs to proudly pursue her hopes and dreams

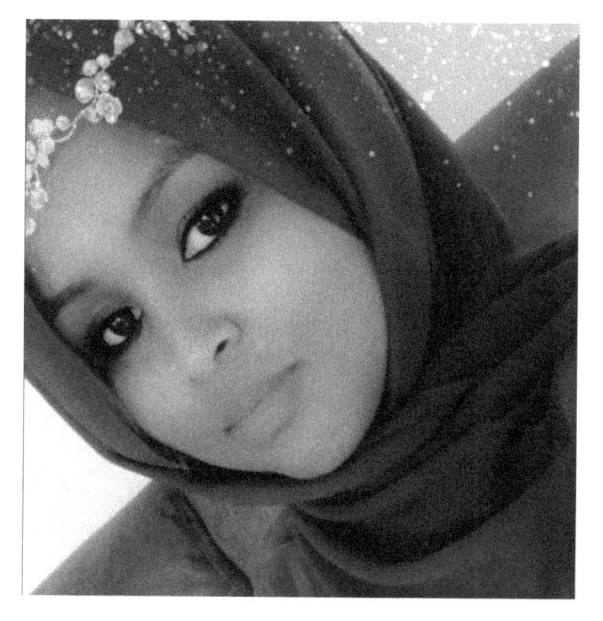

Once feeling alone, worthless and that everyone was judging her, Faduma learned that facing and talking about her pain and challenges was the key to healing. She's now grateful for her blessings and aims to use her difficult journey as a foundation for helping others...

I first experienced depression after I gave birth to my son. I had postnatal depression which is quite common in women. My depression was very severe; I heard voices that constantly told me to take my life.

This started a week after giving birth and I said to myself "you can't tell this to anyone". I feared that if I told healthcare professionals, they would take my baby away. I mean I was thinking of taking my life, I thought *how could I be normal?* I was 22 years old, a mum for the first time and I was a single mother. My circumstances didn't make things easy, in fact they escalated my symptoms.

Healing from the pain of childbirth, I felt as if I was in a war between my body and mind. As the voices got louder, it was hard to know what was real and what was not. I was scared for my son's safety, so if I wasn't feeding him or changing him, he was in his bed. There was no time for bonding. This was survival.

After 2 weeks I realised I wasn't well, and I couldn't continue to live like this, so I told my family. I left my house and stayed with extended family members. Surprisingly the voices weren't there anymore; until this day I believe that house where I heard the voices was haunted. I mean, I didn't hear the voices unless I was inside my house, but as soon as I left they left too.

I decided to move and by the time my son was 6 months old, I found a new place to live. By the will of Allah, our new home felt much safer, and I no longer heard those voices. I started to bond with my baby and started to enjoy being a mother. I still felt depressed every now and then, but not to that extreme length.

Depression came to visit me again when my son got diagnosed with Autism. This time I didn't need voices. I was my own worst enemy. I felt worthless and constantly picked on myself. I was the mother with the sick child. I hated it when people said to me; "May Allah heal your child" because it didn't feel like a dua (prayer), it felt like a statement. I felt like I no longer belonged to my community. I had a disadvantage already for being a single mother, now I had a child with special needs. It was obvious that I didn't have my community's support. I felt like I was just a 'thing' people looked down on, a 'thing' people looked at and thought; *nah I don't want to be associated with her.*

I prayed to Allah asking him for comfort. I cried every day all day. I would look at my son and fear for his future. Would he ever talk? Would he require a lifetime of care? I had so many questions and no one understood my pain. I didn't know who to turn to for comfort, so I turned to food. I ate my feelings and felt guilty the next day. So, I would overeat one day and starve myself the next so I wouldn't get fat. But I started to gain weight. I drove myself to deep depression. I lived inside my head. To the outside world, to my friends and family, I was happy. But they had no idea what was going on inside my head. I started to isolate myself, I felt ugly, fat and worthless. I had to do everything by myself.

This continued for almost 2 years. My son started special school, I was going to uni and working. Things started to feel balanced. But he struggled with sleep, he was up every day at 2am so I'd take him to school, leave my car and take the train, go to uni and sit in a

2 hour lecture half asleep. I couldn't do it. It took a toll on my health big time. I felt the most alone I'd felt in my life.

One day, I decided I was gonna get professional help. I spoke to my GP and was put on antidepressants. It didn't help, they just increased my appetite. So, I did a self referral to Lambeth Talking Therapy. They offered me 6 weeks cognitive behaviour therapy and it was the best decision. I was committed to going to therapy and was honest about how I was feeling. I am still using the techniques I learned during therapy as this isn't a quick fix.

My son is doing well now, he has said his first word, spelled his first word. He is the sweetest little boy and I can't imagine not being his mother. He is a beautiful blessing and I thank Allah for choosing me to be his mother. I am now studying psychology part time and hope one day to be an Educational Psychologist inshallah. I am slowly learning to not be so hard on myself.

I will be 27 this year inshallah and I am glad I didn't listen to those voices and take my life. I have so much to live for and you do too. Never give up.

Ya Allah - Oh God, Al-Ghafoor - the All Forgiving, Ar Raheem - the Most Merciful

Name and attribute of God (Allah)

Sidra is Kinda Proud that she knows herself well enough to make it a superpower

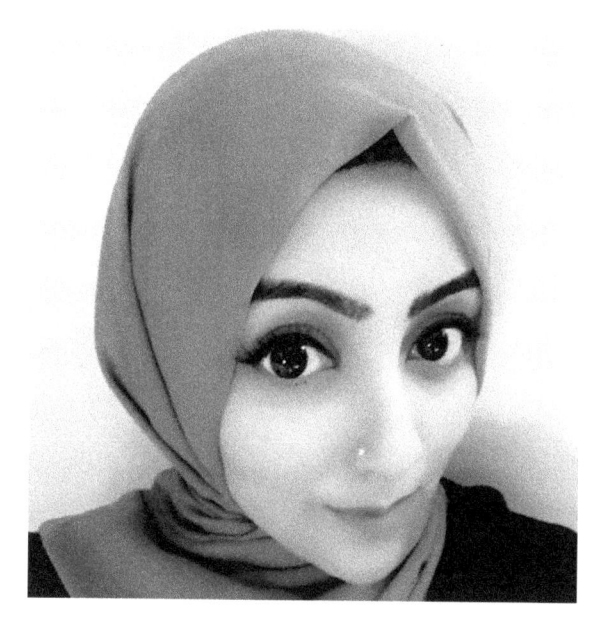

Sidra is now happy to be herself, and so she should be! Her hardships have made her very wise, and she lives life with the healthy concept that, if things don't go the way we think we want them to, then that's because life has a better plan for us. Here Sidra shares the journey that brought her to this belief...

The Journey

Who am I? Is the question I asked myself at different points within my life and today I can say I have found somewhat of an answer; in order for me to tell you that answer I have to take you on a short journey.

1988 born in East London, Muslim, British, Asian, female.

I was brought up as an only child, with wonderful loving parents with unique stories of their own. Teachings from my mother and father shaped me as a person. From a young age I remember sitting with my father listening to stories about Islamic history and stories of the prophets from the Quran.

Sabr (Patience), Hikmah (Wisdom), Tawakkul (Trust in Allah) and Qadr (Decree of Allah) were all part of my life from a very young age and understanding these virtues came about through my upbringing.

1999 Cancer

I remember the day I stood in the corner of the room listening to my father speak after he was told he had cancer "Alhamdulillah it's all with Allah" (thanks be to God) he said. At such a young age I didn't know at the time how these words would shape my life. As the years passed by I witnessed my father's battle against cancer, surgeries, radiotherapy and hospital appointments. I watched as my mother took care of my father; ups and downs of cancer taking its toll at times, yet the one thing that never left my father was his faith and values. Occasionally I felt scared and worried, nevertheless my mother and father always kept me smiling and happy.

2010 - Stroke

We were told half my father's brain had died yet my father lived on but paralysed from one side. Every day I would sit beside his hospital bed, he would write sweet notes to me and my mother. No matter how he changed he was still with us and we were hopeful no matter the hardship.

"Oh what type of life is this? Just like a vegetable", someone once said. I shook with horror and disbelief, this comment affected me deeply. I wanted to scream yet all I could do was keep quiet and cry. The day it all changed *20.06.2010*, on a hot summer's day I kneeled beside my father's hospital bed, his eyes were closed, all tubes had been removed. I gave him a kiss on his forehead, held his hand tight and inside my heart wished I never had to let go, but I knew he was no longer in the land of the living.

Coming home from the mosque after my father was buried, grief hit me like a stormy ocean wave, drowning me, unable to breathe. All I could do was cry. My hero was gone. I was lost and felt so alone. "He's gone, just accept it", someone said "get a grip, he's watching, you're making his soul sad", another told us. At the time of my grief I was unable to eat and lost 9kg in two weeks, I felt I was unable to move forward. Comments people made added to my pain and I was unable to push them aside as it took me time to understand the needs of my mind and body. Grief comes in many different forms and lack of understanding and labels can cause dire mental health issues.

2017- Accepting an illness

Keratoconus is a non-inflammatory eye condition in which the normally dome shape of the eye (the cornea) changes shape, causing vision to decrease and in severe cases causing blindness.

The time I was told I had the illness, I remembered my father's words "Alhamdulillah for everything", I said. You see, my mother also suffers from Keratoconus and growing up I watched her struggle. When she arrived in England in the 1970s she became a patient at Moorfield eye Hospital. Due to the lack of early care my mother became partially sighted, unable to see without hard contact lenses. August 2017 I had cross linking surgery on both eyes; this was extremely painful and traumatising. The healing process was lengthy, I had to stay in a dark room for four months, unable to see clearly for one year, having to deal with the pain and scarring within my eyes.

Accepting I have this illness was a major challenge in my life. The fear of not being able to see overtook my thoughts at times. I felt sadness and slowly accepted that my vision will decrease over the years. Here again I faced labels, labels that people put on me. Comments made in passing, without the thought of how it would affect me.

The Journey of learning

Who am I? Fear or challenge, uncertainty or opportunity, anxiety or excitement, Sabr, Hikmah, Tawakkul and Qadr. Labels and words have always affected me, the lack of kindness or understanding in words can affect us all unknowingly. Addressing this can be a challenge within itself, however in not doing so we only affect our own mental health. I found having an open respectful conversation with Hikmah of speaking we can address and challenge the labels that others place on us. I have found positivity in having awareness of myself, placing healthy boundaries and growing as a person. When thinking about something negative I now try to counteract it with something positive. The days I feel overwhelmed by my emotions and thoughts, I now embrace them rather than suppressing them. It is okay to not be okay and own it. Our 'imperfections' make us who we are, and we are all beautiful regardless of words and comments.

> *"No one is you and that is your superpower"*
> Dave Grohl

In our lives we all have been in situations where we have no control; death of loved ones, illnesses and uncertainties in life. It's okay to be honest about how you feel, what you're experiencing and what you need or want. It is important to understand your own mind and body, to not push yourself and accept the things about yourself you might dislike.

Over the years I have found peace in Tawakkul, if you did not get something you want or something did not go your way, know that Allah has something better planned for you. Alhumdulillah ala kulli haal (All praises are for Allah in every condition). I found that stories from the Quran helped me accept struggles within my life, understanding Qadr and having Sabr, helped me overcome my sadness of loss and accepting my illness. We go through life not understanding why bad things happen to us but when we change our perspective, knowing there is a higher plan in everything that happens, we come to a self-understanding, a deeper understanding of our own hearts. Today I am thankful to Allah for every hardship put in my path as there is Hikmah behind every test and I feel I am who I am because of every test I faced.

Through my experiences regarding my father and through his values I want to live a life of meaning, leaving behind a legacy by helping others with their hardships.

> *"Verily with hardship comes ease"*
> Qur'an Surah Ash-Sharh, 94:6

> *"Do not lose hope, nor be sad"*
> Qur'an Surah Ali 'Imran, 3:139

I've learnt to overcome my hardship with the right tools, everyone's tools are different and we each have our own stories. No one's way of feeling pain is wrong, it's all about how we deal with that pain which defines a person. Self-love is knowing your worth, being kind to yourself, embracing who you are and forgiving yourself for your shortcomings.

Who am I? I am me and I am happy being me.

Sidra Katib

"Al-Mujib - The One who answers all"
Name and attribute of God (Allah)

Sophia, Part 2: Post- Pandemic Growth

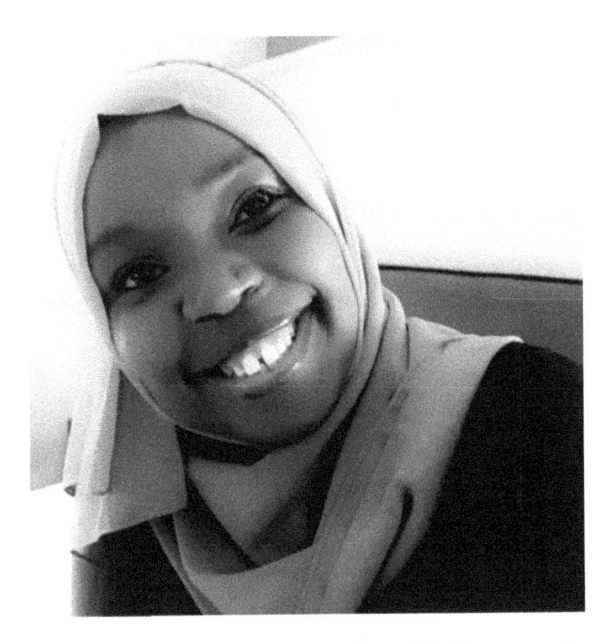

Since we started discussions as the publishing team for this pocket book project before the Covid-19 pandemic hit, all of the team have experienced big life transitions over the last year and it therefore made sense to share some of these shifts and learnings at the end of the book.

Here Sophia shares the next stage of her painful journey of being forced to STOP, surrender and continue learning as the pandemic arrived to impact her life…

The journey of life is like a fast train, going in and out of tunnels: we and everyone around us has our own individual stop. For some of us we don't get off the fast train until something forces us to stop. This heeding comes in different forms, whether it's trauma, a physical illness, hiccups in life or an overwhelming sense of anxiety about life itself. I am sure there are many more reasons that others have experienced this, which I have not been able to mention. My personal force came in the form of the pandemic: the dreaded lockdown, the anxiety of the uncertainty contained in it all, and the world coming to a halt.

The Covid-19 pandemic trickled down its avalanche into the world causing so much devastation and loss. It hit hard, it almost brought me to my knees, and I had to redefine the ideas I had created in my head about life and my recovery. I lost all of my coping mechanisms and I felt stripped from everything I had worked so hard for during my therapy years. Even the self-help books that I had collected and invested in throughout the years were not helping me. My anxiety reached a record high level, a level that I'd never experienced before. I became scared of death. I feared losing my loved ones and I found myself crying almost every day and desperately watching the news and reading stories, hoping to have a sense of an end to the pandemic. Conversations around family became increasingly difficult, and I felt somewhat disconnected from everything, everyone and even myself.

During these days I would find myself crying about the loss of thousands of people dying from Covid-19. Then, suddenly, I felt like I was grieving the death of my father all over again. This time my grief focused on how he'd died, the way he was killed. The murder itself, the individuals that were involved.

My heart was aching, I wanted and demanded answers. But there was no one I felt I could turn to, to answer all of the questions that were running through my head. Why did they kill him? I tried to bury everything I was feeling, and I became mute once again. Thoughts were racing through my head, but I did not dare to whisper a word to anyone. I felt ashamed to still be grieving my father's death as it was so many years ago, but the pause in our lives had forced me to face the pain that was simmering deep inside me. One of my addictions was to keep busy, working all of the time: if I was not working then I was studying something deep and intense. All this I now realise was to escape my feelings and the reality of my pain...

Father's Day Poem

To him who I never got to know, or hug, or tell him how much he is missed every day!

This one day dedicated in your name cannot justify a daughter's love for her absent father.

All the missed first days have become dried tears, my graduation, when mum said you would be proud, what about my wedding day where you never got to give me away?...

For all the daughters and sons, waking up with a heavy heart, for the fathers whose children do not value their worth, to my mother and all of the women who played my father's role, you are so loved!

May Allah mend all the broken hearts of absent love that never got to blossom…

I started revisiting old habits of suffering in silence, but I had another battle to fight. I started experiencing severe symptoms of Carpal Tunnel Syndrome (CTS). My hands felt like they were burning and hammered down. Electric shocks started from my shoulder and travelled all the way down to my fingertips. The symptoms began only at night, but then they started every minute of every day during the lockdown. One afternoon the pain was so unbearable that I started to think the worst. Doctors were not seeing patients, and everything was shut down. I felt trapped and suffered a range of emotions. Even after explaining to family and friends, no one around me knew what CTS was. For them my hands looked normal, no injury, no broken bones so they could not understand why I was in so much pain. It reminded me a lot of when we suffer mental distress and because it cannot be seen and sometimes not heard, our loved ones struggle to understand the impact it has on us.

Emotional Pain

Emotional Pain

Cannot be seen...

Cannot be heard...

Sometimes it is ignored

But it paralyses you

Comes to your silent hours

When the world sleeps, yours is awake...

Emotional pain

Lies deeper than the scars,

Deep beneath the seeping wounds,

Emotional Pain

Takes longer to heal

But it is worth beginning the process

Do not let your pain overwhelm your soul

When you are ready someone is waiting to take your hand and walk beside you through this emotional journey.

Once again, I started to hear the same advice I have heard before; "go to a spiritual healer, you are doomed if you do not, this must be the evil eye". I felt suffocated, almost like I could not breathe. I started to open up to my best friend and my sister, I started to express how I was feeling. The physical pain felt easier to describe. Still, I could not express my grief and how I was feeling about my father's death.

We started to read up about CTS and I was able to match all of the symptoms that I was reading about to the ones I was experiencing.

Then one day, my friend found me on the floor crying, I felt so overwhelmed. I started opening up about my father and the anger I was feeling. I started reading stories of other families whose loved ones had been killed. I started turning to Allah (God) and seeking guidance through my prayers. My sister suggested I try to go to a private treatment about my CTS, so I came across a consultant who was a specialist in CTS. This is how my journey of physical and emotional healing began.

I started therapy again and I knew that I could take my pain safely to my therapist. After every session I had a good cry and felt like something in me was starting to let go of all the negative emotions. I started talking about my father and I started to understand that I never really gave myself time to grieve and that grief itself came in so many different emotions. For me it was denial, I was still waiting for him to appear one day and that the news about his death had been mistaken identity. Not attending his funeral did not give me a chance to say goodbye and those feelings of never being able to meet him again paralysed me. For me accepting the loss, my loss that Dad was gone and, in this life, I was never going to see him again. I started to accept this, and I started to let go, and I placed my hope in meeting him, one day, on the other side.

After months of being on the waiting list, I had surgery for my CTS. The first night I came back home from the hospital I slept like a baby. The first sound sleep that I had in almost a year. It is amazing what sleep can do for the mind and body. I also recognised this because my CTS caused nerve pain: all those negative emotions that I was carrying around, buried deep inside, must have escalated the physical pain I had, and it was unbearable.

I found my stop on this fast train that I was on, and although the halt for me was the lockdown, it forced me to work on the underlying issues. The source of my pain, not just on the surface but on the inside too.

Alhamdullilah (thanks be to God) I sought His guidance and His help, and I was open to whatever form it came in. I was desperate to continue my healing and I know that I have some way to go, but I am back on the journey.

Reflection...

When I am in pain, I often think about...

What does Allah want me to learn from this?

When the pain is too deep... I supplicate...

Al-Jabbar -The Compeller, The Restorer

(Ya Jabbar mend my broken heart)

"oh Allah, Al Aleem (The All-Knowing) teach me..."

We know that in everything good or bad, there is a lesson.

"And your Lord says, "Call upon Me: I will respond to you."
Qur'an, Surah Ghafir, 40:60

Ayan, Part 2: A Dedication to Self and Others

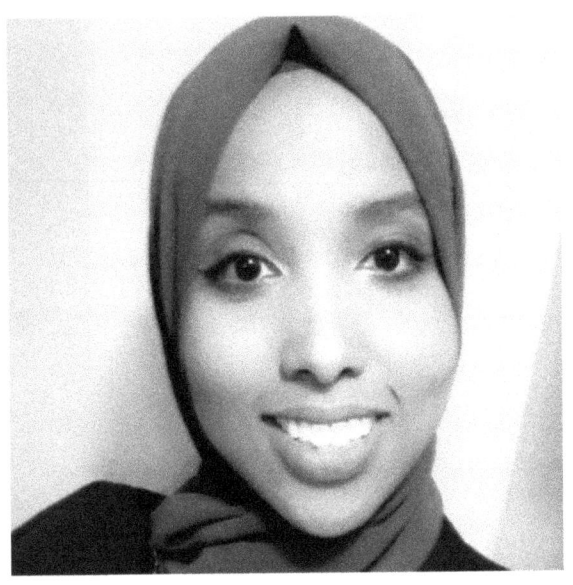

Along with team member Sophia, the experience of living through the last year of the Covid-19 pandemic has taken its toll on Ayan. But rather than let the challenges drag her back into mental distress, she's learned to become the observer of her emotions and utilise them as an opportunity for personal growth.

We love the woman Ayan has become, full of wisdom, empathy, compassion, hopes and dreams. But more importantly, so does she…

I continue to suffer, learn, and change. Healing is an ongoing journey.

This is part 2 of my story. It is striking to see how much your life can change in a year or two.

Life itself is a journey that must be travelled despite how unpleasant the road might be. I am learning to trust the journey even though I may not understand it sometimes. The reality is that not everyone will understand your journey, especially if they have never walked a similar path.

My path to spiritual awakening mainly began in my mid 20's. It stemmed from my traumatic experience of spiritual abuse by a fake 'spiritual healer' in 2012, as mentioned in part 1 of my story. Allow me to explain further how this person abused his position. Not only did he electrocute my hands whilst reciting some verses from the Quran, but he also made me drink something and smell a particular scent. He asked for my full name, my mother's name. He was verbally abusive, claiming that he was talking to the evil spirit that was inside me. I recall a moment when he would ask me to call upon someone other than Allah, which I remember refusing because it is Shirk. I recollect how I kept repeating the Shahada, which is the Muslim declaration of faith that expresses the belief that "There is no God but Allah and that Muhammad is the messenger of Allah".

Although not diagnosed, I experienced CPTSD (complex post-traumatic stress disorder) symptoms many years after this spiritual abuse. During this time, I fell in and out of experiencing depression, anxiety and symptoms that could not have been medically explained. Until today, at times I experience flashbacks, dreams, electricity sensations, even suddenly smelling the scent he made me smell. A decade later, my knowledge and understanding of mental health and life, in general, is entirely different.

Looking back, I can now say this significant event in my life was like a re-birth event to my authentic self. I started waking up to connect with my authentic self reasonably late in life, but I guess it is better late than never. My journey to self-growth began when I started to look for reasons for my mental health distress.

I have been on a healing journey, and I was fascinated to find answers to my pain and address it at many different levels. It almost felt like I was on a mission to "cure" myself, or at least live a more fulfilling life full of inner peace and contentment. I went through the internal conflict of understanding the cause of my suffering and how I could be 'cured'? Which now, looking back on this itself, caused me anxiety. As a Muslim, my family was adamant that the cause of my suffering was black magic or the evil eye, and I understood that it was both mental health distress and some elements of the afflictions of spiritual issues. I always make dua (supplication) to Allah (God) to help me understand his Qadr (decree), not just to 'understand', but for guidance, manifestation and Allah to bless me with Hikmah (wisdom).

As part of my healing journey, I found somewhat of an answer.

I was fortunate to participate in a 12-week course in 2019 run by Dr Sara Betteridge from the BME Access service in East London Foundation Trust, held in the Maryam centre East London mosque. The main course content included the Qalb (Spiritual Heart), the Aql (Ability to reason) & the Nafs (Soul), how they function, how to nurture them and how to protect them. Understanding mental health, the impact it has on the heart, mind, and soul. Psychological approaches to dealing with mental health complement Islamic approaches.

As a person who experienced childhood and adulthood complex trauma, I have not come across any Islamic institute or organisation that brings these two approaches together, providing a holistic approach for Muslims. Throughout the 12 weeks, I felt connected and confident that my life was not just empty rituals.

Even though I had a brief understanding at the time, what struck me on the course was the concept of CBT (cognitive behavioural therapy), understanding thoughts and emotions and thus our behaviours. How we view ourselves dictates how we see and interpret the world. I recognised that negative self-perception might also dictate a negative perception of Allah.

I recall feeling empty, lonely and hostile about who I was. Looking back now, I believe this was due to the lack of a sense of Self. When I know myself and live aligned to my values and beliefs, I have strong connections to myself and others, and I have passion, drive, purpose, and life feels full and worth living. However, in 2011-2016, I lacked a sense of Self which led to the opposite. When I did not know who I was as an individual, my mood, purpose and goals drastically varied with my changing circumstances.

It was a profound introductory course that increased a deeper level to my relationship with Allah (God) and my relationship with myself. I gained many insights, and one of them is knowing that Islam as a faith is very much a heart-centred one. As a Muslim, I found the holistic approach in understanding and bringing together western psychology and the Islamic perspective of the 'Self' to be a life-changing experience.

Trauma

This section is so dear to my heart, and at times challenging to process. It took me months to write it up. You see, trauma is not about the sinister events that happen to us but rather what happens inside us due to the traumatic events. Trauma lies on a continuum, and it looks different for people because we all have different lived experiences. When it comes to mental, emotional, spiritual and physical distress, we often think, what is wrong with people instead of what has happened to them? What is their story?

Carrying childhood trauma might trigger other adulthood trauma, and throughout my life, this has caused me to disconnect from my true authentic Self. Trauma tends to disconnect us from our feelings, body, and sometimes to the world around us, to the point I went through dissociative experiences.

When I experienced pain in my childhood, the pain was there, and I had no one to share it with. This was due to many reasons, simply because I was just a child and not knowing what was done to me had been wrong. Also, from the trauma event being normalised to be something done culturally or even to the point that religion is used to justify it, when now in my adult life having done my research, it is far from what Islam promotes. Another childhood traumatic incident I experienced again involved not understanding what was done to me was abuse. It came with 'shame' that I carried throughout my life, thinking it happened because I allowed it to happen. Shame (Ceeb in the Somali language) is a killer for childhood traumas. I carried this experience with me subconsciously and recently kept saying to myself, "if only I would put up a fight if only I had run away if only I have done this/that".

Reflecting on this, I do not think I got traumatised because I was wronged, but I got traumatised because I was alone with my hurt.

Taking my pain to therapy has been extremely difficult but yet rewarding at the same time. I recognised that there was a strong link between my spiritual abuse and my childhood trauma experiences. It was clear and made total sense why I tended to experience postpartum depression every time I gave birth. When I made these trauma connections, it opened another door to healing. Through self-work and therapy, I realised the importance of re-parenting my inner child alongside parenting my two princesses, having self-kindness and self-compassion.

The awareness of my traumas was essential because once I understood it, especially the complex childhood trauma, it made me more compassionate to myself as I was just a child and did not have the right help or support. When we start the journey of being compassionate with ourselves, not only does it change us, our children, our families, it changes communities and the broader society at large.

It is not the question of just getting rid of these childhood trauma memories, as I feel my experiences have been invalidated, and many loved ones have told me, "it is in the past; forget about it and move on". I wish it were that easy. Do you think people choose to keep their traumatic memories and want to suffer in life?

We need to see people beyond their trauma and pain. Yes, sure, our life experiences shape us for who we are today. However, just because I choose to voice myself and help anyone that experiences mental or emotional distress, it certainly does not mean that my trauma and lived experience define who I am.

I am now fortunate to have gained self-awareness, tools to aid me in being connected to the real me by re-learning my values and beliefs, shaping my identity and the ideal person I want to become.

I do not see myself as a 'victim' to my past traumatic experiences anymore.

People who have experienced trauma often represent their life as being single-storied. I was living a life as if I was trapped in a single dimension of my life, one that promoted a sense of shame, despair, depression, emptiness and hopelessness. Through my studies and lived experience, I learned that we do not respond to what happens to us in life, but we react to our perception of what happens. It is with our minds that we create the world.

Yes, I still feel anxious or have low moods here and there, but healing comes with something inside of me that is constantly changing for the good. Part of that could be the 'shame' I carried due to my childhood trauma, spiritual abuse, or mental distress itself is slowly dissipating. When we connect to the fact that the source of change is within us, we gain agency and learn that we have self-autonomy and the power to make positive changes in our lives. The beauty of healing is that once I started to reframe things, re-author or re-story my life, through this book, through therapy, through meaningful conversations with different people that supported me. I began to live my preferred way of life.

I learned and Changed....

Covid-19 – Grief and Loss

2020 has been a year of testing for everyone, as the world shared the experience of the global trauma of the Pandemic. It highlighted for me a verse in the Quran, Surah Baqarah (chapter 2), verse 155, where Allah (God) says, *"And certainly, we shall test you with something of fear, hunger, loss of wealth, lives and fruits, but give glad tidings to As-Saabiroon (the patient)."* I remember I kept thinking what this verse meant for me, and it made me realise that as much as we as human beings do not like the suffering of pain or loss of any kind, it is inevitable.

Like any life event, the pandemic came with its positives, bringing communities and the world together. However, it also came with unpleasant experiences, such as the death of loved ones, grief, loss of jobs, domestic violence and the rise of mental and emotional distress.

During these uncertain times, I was fortunate to get a promotion in the NHS as a Senior Peer Support worker. I started a postgraduate/ master's course in Integrative Counselling and Coaching with the University of East London. Studying during the pandemic had its challenging moments. Still, it has granted me hope and patience as it reminded me to treasure life, loved ones, and my ultimate passion for helping others.

However, I faced many personal challenges during this period. I was stuck at home, wearing many hats, such as working part-time while homeschooling and studying. I was not just experiencing anxiety through distorted cognition, but I also experienced it as bodily sensations daily, which I could not seem to switch off from. What helped me was going for a walk, usually with a friend or alone, whilst listening to personal, self-work or spiritual development podcasts.

Many of the psychological theories I have learnt assisted me in persevering in my studies and becoming a better person. I benefitted from having personal therapy, which has made me reflect on how difficult it has been for me in doing self-work on my own. It helps when you have someone alongside you on your journey who listens, validates and makes you feel heard. It is that simple; people yearn for a safe space, where they feel listened to, heard, validated, not judged for their lived experiences. They have their answers and solutions within them.

I acknowledged how resilient I was as a person, despite going through anxiety, grief, the loss of close relationships, dealing with feelings of not being good enough as a trainee therapist, self-doubt, imposter syndrome, inadequacies and incompetence.

I used to associate grief with losing someone through death, but I have come to learn that it is more than that. Grief is a natural process that our body goes through after the experience of any loss. Reflecting on the spiritual abuse I encountered, it was a loss of self-identity that I experienced. Unfortunately, I never knew how to grieve, and it just built up. This could be due to the way I have been conditioned growing up. In my culture, I have always been taught to act strong and move on.

I found the grief of the relationship breakdown of some family members and friends at different times during the pandemic very difficult to deal with. I realised that time is too precious to play around with negative people. So, I mustered up the courage to part ways with a few of them. Cutting people out of my life is never easy, but I found I was much better off for having done it. I learned that taking time away from friends, some families, setting boundaries for relationships, and stepping away from drama does not make you the wrong person. It is great to be a support system for your friends, but it is equally important that I take care of my mental health and my own needs in the process. With distance and self-reflection, I felt a lot calmer and ready to apologise sincerely on my behalf. I learnt to take time out to take some deep breaths and become conscious of my thinking. Distancing helped provide space and give me time to self-reflect and gain a complete picture of a situation.

However, it hit me that I was cutting people off left, right, and centre. I started to look within and realised all the people I had to cut off in my life had many things in common. It was an awakening for me to look deeper and go inward by looking at where I contributed and where I was going wrong in repeating similar relationship patterns.

One of the key learnings for me was again my relationship with setting boundaries. Until today I often find it difficult and uncomfortable in setting boundaries. I explored further and recognised that I was suffering from people-pleasing and codependency. Codependency is usually rooted in childhood, and codependent relationships are a response to unaddressed past traumas. I was raised in a home, a culture where emotions were ignored or even punished. When certain older family members felt a feeling, we all shared it. This phenomenon of codependency still blows my mind. With all the things I have been through and conquered, I still have to manage this default behaviour pattern I learned in my childhood. Recovering from codependency is one of the trickiest parts of healing. I constantly find myself adapting to others' moods, trying to please or not upset anyone, fearing being disliked or abandoned if I set a boundary.

I experienced feelings of confusion and disappointment due to the fallout with some family and friends. I felt hurt and taken back by what they did and their use of words. The more I pushed away from these uncomfortable feelings, the more intense it became. Therefore, accepting it for what it is was my first step. The interventions that supported me and made me feel at peace were mindfulness and daily prayers. The Islamic daily prayers, I see as a form of meditation, it helped me look within and accept myself for who I am. After my meditation and making duas (supplications), by talking to Allah (God) about the deep pain of my heart, using his beautiful name '*Al-Wadud*' (the most loving), I often felt a sense of peace and contentment. When I am at ease, I tend to have unconditional positive regard for myself, self-compassion, and others whenever I fall short.

I feel like I am more conscious now in my life than I have ever been. I am a lot less anxious, and I enjoy taking things slowly, taking care of myself mentally, emotionally and spiritually, and having self-compassion.

Self-awareness allows me to keep an eye on my inner as well as my external world. Although it requires effort and time, it can be powerful and valuable in many ways. I usually find it helpful in having meaningful conversations and expressing myself. Self-disclosure and showing vulnerability have helped enhance self-awareness and genuinely finding my authentic Self. Knowing myself and having self-awareness helps with connecting with my feelings and emotions. Understanding the difference between feelings and emotions gives me more choices and more control of my behaviour.

You see, new grief experiences trigger older unaddressed, unprocessed grief experiences. I learnt that there is a difference between experiencing grief and processing grief. I think grief hits us inside and is an energy that we may not know what to do with. The part of processing grief I found helpful was allowing the feelings (which were extreme at the moment) to pass through me. When I allowed these feelings, I reflected on what emotions came up for me, and it helped when I named it and accepted it for what it was. My experience of grief made me realise that grief does not come with just a single emotion, but rather it comes with many strong feelings and emotions simultaneously, such as sadness, hurt, despair, and rejection.

Being aware of my emotions and dealing with them by properly channelling them aids me to be an emotionally healthy person.

I do not think emotions and feelings are negative or positive. Society and cultures make us put them in boxes. I believe it is part of human nature to experience these emotions.

Emotions and feelings are signals.

I think of them as messengers helping me move through the world in a responsive and integrated manner. I approach it now by welcoming and listening to them rather than getting rid of them.

The Quran very clearly shows us that feeling our emotions is a foundational step to vulnerability. I believe that in the Muslim community, we need to stop incorrectly correlating complicated feelings with ingratitude. Someone can be feeling intense pain and still be grateful. We see this with the examples of all Prophets. A great example of this is in the story of Yusuf, Chapter 12 in the Quran. Prophet Yusuf's father, Prophet Yaqub, when he suffered the loss of his son, Yusuf, and his eyesight, Prophet Yacub says, "I complain of my anguish and grief to Allah" (Quran 12:86). The prophets did not hide from their emotional states, so why should you and I?

The names and attributes of Allah I have chosen to share in this book that has kept me alive even when I felt like I had no one that understood, heard, listened or validated me are *As-Samee* 'The All-Hearing", *Al-Baseer* "The All-Seeing" and *Al-Aleem* "The All-Knowing".

Allah (God) tells us throughout the Quran that He is *As-Samee*, *Al-Baseer*! He is the All-Hearing, the All-Seeing. I opened my heart and let myself be sufficed by Him seeing me and hearing me.

Humans can fail me. However, there is such great power in being seen and heard by my creator, who knows me better than I know myself. Regardless of what I am going through, where I am at or how I feel, just knowing that I am always under Allah's love and His watchful eye gives me Hope. My grief and tears in this world are heard and seen. My story, my past, my struggles from the day I was born until now, my hopes and dreams, the words I do not share with anyone, the heartbreak that feels heavy to carry, my efforts have all been heard and seen by Him.

He is *Al-Aleem*, "The All-Knowing".

I want to share my story hoping that I might return that small place of refuge to someone else. Right now, some people suffer in silence with their mental and emotional distress, trying to figure out how to receive love, and we as a society tell them they are "too much."

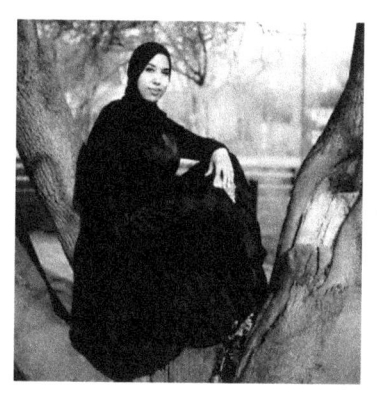

I was fortunate to be one of the nominees for the Women's Inclusive Team, International Women's day 2021 wall of fame.

Despite the grief, I was experiencing it at the time of this picture. I am still astonished at how I have shown up, represented, and inspired women and created HOPE.

My grief experience, mental health distress does NOT define me. My resilience to continue serving myself and others even though my struggles exist is what defines me.

I have had the opportunity to get to know myself on a deeper level, and I am forever grateful to Allah for all experiences, for indeed, there is always good in Allah's Qadr. It may be challenging, bitter and complex while in hardship but there is always ease that comes with it.

I long for a place where we could be more open about the dysfunctional history most of us share and believe we should have an open dialogue that is not drenched in shame of our lived experiences of mental and emotional distress.

My hope for the future is to create safe spaces where mental health distress is normalised, breaking the silence and stigma around mental health issues. My lifelong goal is to set up an organisation to work with the community by counselling individuals and provide coaching sessions.

My journey has taken years, tears, and hours of reflection and mindfulness, and I hope my story can bring freedom to others and the knowledge that they are not alone. I have been granted some of the most gracious companions that life has to offer, who had treated me with the delicacy and love I needed when I was suffering the most.

This is dedicated to them.

Resources for Muslims struggling with mental distress

Crisis Helplines, Text and Web services - UK

Samaritans National Lifeline UK & Ireland:

116 123 (UK & Ireland) | Email jo@samaritans.org

Whatever you're going through, call the Samaritans free anytime, from any phone on **116 123**. There is someone there to answer the phone 24 hours a day, 365 days a year. This number is **FREE** to call. You don't have to be suicidal to call the Samaritans.

In an emergency: Call **999** – If you or someone else is in immediate risk of serious harm or injury you should call the emergency services.

Contact your GP – if you, a friend or relative is experiencing mental health problems.

Muslim Women's Helpline – Phone: **0800 999 5786** (free from mobiles and landlines) 10am to 4pm (Mon to Fri) **0741 520 6936** (Usual call rates apply)

Text: **07415 206 936** - Will respond during operating hours

Mind Helpline – open 24hrs everyday **0121 262 3555** (or Freephone **0800 915 9292**)

Please note: Whilst the Resources information in this pocket book is considered to be true and correct at the date of publication, changes post publication may impact on the accuracy of the information supplied above. Please check online for up to date contact numbers if you are in distress and in need of support.

Below we have provided helpful links to organisations that have a series of free resources to help improve mental wellbeing which you will be able to read online or download. Please note we do not hold any affiliation with any particular organisation or recommend any specifically, this list is intended purely as a guide to what we have found to be helpful.

The Yaqeen Institute for Islamic Research is dedicated to the publication of original content, on relevant Islamic topics, that is academic, authentic, and accessible. Yaqeen Institute has a section that provides research on trauma and adversity from a psychospiritual perspective and theoretical and empirical research on the psychological processes involved in belief, doubt, and religious identity:

https://yaqeeninstitute.org/read/psychology-mental-health

Contact: info@yaqeeninstitute.org

Inspirited Minds is a faith based, grassroots mental health charity located in London that launched in 2014 with the aim to raise awareness, combat stigmas and provide professional, non-judgemental, confidential support to those with mental health issues:

www.inspiritedminds.org.uk

Muslim Youth helpline are a faith and culturally sensitive support by phone, live chat, Whatsapp or email who offer non-judgemental, confidential support 7 days a week, 365 days a year including bank holidays and Eid:

Muslim Youth Helpline 7 days a week (4pm-10pm)
0808 808 2008

https://myh.org.uk

Muslim Counsellor and Psychotherapist Network (MCAPN) is the online platform where you can find Muslim Counsellors, Psychotherapists, Psychiatrists and Counselling Psychologists locally or worldwide:

www.mcapn.co.uk

Sakoon are providers of Islamic Counselling Services in the UK with clients worldwide:

www.Sakoon.co.uk
Telephone: 07943 561 561
email: info@sakoon.co.uk

MindworksUK is a service provider to local charities and companies primarily within South London and other London boroughs. Due to the pandemic they are now accepting referrals outside of London. All of their face to face sessions have currently reverted to using Zoom or telephone sessions or a similar platform:

www.mindworksuk.co.uk

Approachable Parenting offer a variety of services and courses, which link modern Psychological theory and coaching techniques to the Muslim faith. You can contact them and leave a message on the landline: 0121-7738643, they will pick up your message and respond.

Alternatively, you can send an email to info@approachableparenting.org.uk:

www.Approachableparenting.org

Self-Care Tips

"Those who believe, and whose hearts find satisfaction in the remembrance of Allah: for without doubt in the remembrance of Allah do hearts find satisfaction."
Qur'an, Surah Ar-Ra'd, 13:28

A crisis is different for everyone, but one thing is the same for all of us: when we are in a crisis we can feel as though everything is falling apart.

These tips aim to give you some simple but vital tools that can help you to stay safe and manage your thoughts and feelings.

Having our experiences validated as 'normal', real, natural and meaningful can be one of the most important aspects of being able to heal and grow.

It's vital that we are kind to ourselves during this time, and allow any emotions to surface and be expressed in a safe environment.

Having peer support from someone who has gone through similar experiences, and can listen without judgement, is really helpful. Go to the resources section to find services that may be most helpful for you personally.

You are not alone! What you are going through is a normal part of a healing process. Don't give up – there is a light at the end of the tunnel, even when you feel in complete darkness.

You are not crazy, the healing journey is a painful process, but one well worth embarking on.

Quick Tips to keep yourself safe:

- Remember that your thoughts do not have to take charge - you can have them without acting on them

- If you are feeling like hurting yourself, wait, even if it's for 5 minutes, but just wait, and breathe slow and deep…This may be hard but it's likely the intensity will subside

- Call a person or group you can trust to open up to about how you feel

- Find a safe environment e.g. with a therapist or in a group, to help you work through trauma when it arises to be healed. Releasing your emotions - verbally, physically and in any other way necessary - is vital

- Find a safe way to express any emotions that are surfacing

- Focus on your self-care - Getting physical exercise / being in nature / eating wholesome food and getting plenty of sleep is important. Initially, some prescribed medications may be necessary to help you manage your life

- Avoid stimulants (alcohol / drugs / caffeine / processed foods, especially sugar)

- Join a support group – this can be an online forum, it helps not to isolate yourself. Try to find at least one person you trust who you can openly talk to about your experiences without fear of being judged

- Listening to calming sounds or the sounds of nature can be helpful

- Relationships - spend time with supportive people, and distance yourself from ones that feel stressful

- Creative self-expression is helpful when you find talking difficult, e.g. drawing, painting, poetry, music, drumming, sculpture, singing

- Call a helpline and talk about how you feel, e.g. the Samaritans (look in the Resources section to find one that feels right for you)

Prayers in the morning and the evening:

Some of the most frequent supplications that the Prophet would make are those commonly referred to as supplications of the morning and evening. The "morning" here refers to the time between dawn (fajr) and sunrise, while the "evening" refers to the beginning of 'asr time until sunset. Below are a few that we have chosen for the purpose of this book, please see the www.islamhashtag.com/fortress-of-muslim-pdf/ for the full version of the morning and evening supplications.

Morning Du'ā

Asbahnā wa-asbaha al-mulku lillāhi wa-al-hamdu lillāhi lā ilāha illā Allāhu wahdahu lā sharīka lahu, lahu al-mulku wa-lahu al-hamdu wa-huwa 'alá kulli shay'in qadīr. Rabbi as'aluka khayra mā fī hādhā al-yawmi wa-khayra mā ba'dahu wa-a'ūdhu bika min sharri mā fī hādhā al-yawmi wa-sharri mā ba'dah. Rabbi a'ūdhu bika min al-kasali wa-sū' al-kibari rabbi a'ūdhu bika min 'adhābin fī al-nāri wa-'adhābin fī al-qabr.

Translation: We have reached the morning, and all sovereignty remains with Allah this morning, and all praise is for Allah. There is no true God except Allah, alone, without a partner. To Him belongs all sovereignty and praise and He has power over all things. My Lord, I ask You for the good in this day and the good of what follows it, and I seek refuge in You from the evil in this day and the evil of what follows it. My Lord, I seek refuge in You from laziness and from the harms of old age. My Lord, I seek refuge in You from torment in the Fire and punishment in the grave. [Muslim]

Allāhumma innī as'aluka al-'āfiyah fī al-dunyá wa-al-ākhirah allāhumma innī as'aluka al-'afwah wa-al-'āfiyah fī dīnī wa-dunyāya wa-ahlī wa-mālī allāhumma ustur 'awrātī wa-āmin raw'ātī allāhumma ihfaznī min bayni yadayya wa-min khalfī wa-'an yamīnī wa-'an shimālī wa-min fawqī wa-a'ūdhu bi-'azamatika an ughtāla min tahtī.

Translation: O Allah, I ask You for well-being in this world and the Hereafter. O Allah, I ask You for pardon and well-being in my religion, my worldly affairs, my family and my property. O Allah, conceal my faults and keep me safe from what I fear. O Allah, guard me from in front of me and behind me, on my right and on my left, and from above me. And I seek refuge in Your Magnificence from being swallowed up from beneath me.

[Abū Dāwud and Ibn Mājah]

Evening Du'ā

A'ūdhu bi-kalimāti Allāhi al-tāmmāti min sharri mā khalaq.

Translation: I seek refuge in the Perfect Words of Allah from the evil of what He has created.
(Hadith Muslim)

Context: Abū Hurayrah reported that a person came to the prophet Muhammad Peace and Blessings be Upon Him (Pbuh) and said, "Allah's Messenger, I was stung by a scorpion last night." The Prophet (Pbuh) said, "Had you recited these words in the evening: 'I seek refuge in the Perfect Words of Allah from the evil of what He has created,' it would not have harmed you."

[Hadith Muslim 2709]

All citations have been sited in Prophetic Prayers for Relief and Protection | Yaqeen Institute for Islamic Research by Dr. Tahir Wyatt *Director of Systematic Theology, Associate Editor- April 2020.*

Many of the contributors have found contemplating and reflecting on the 99 names of Allah to be highly beneficial when going through mental distress of any kind:

www.99namesofallah.name/download-99-names-of-allah/

Suicidal thoughts and Self-Harm

Even though a crisis can be growth towards healing, there may be times when it is extremely dark, terrifying, and dangerous; it is common to experience having suicidal thoughts and thoughts of self-harm.

There are, however, a lot of things that can help manage this distress, more of which can be found on this link:

www.youngminds.org.uk/find-help/feelings-and-symptoms/suicidal-feelings/

The fact is you are not alone: other people have felt deep and terrible pain and come through it and you can too.

Feeling suicidal does not have to mean giving up on life.

If you are feeling suicidal it may be that you are desperate for things to be different. Wanting this life to end doesn't rule out the possibility of a new, better life beginning, but you may feel like that is beyond reach right now. Imagine what a better life might look like and see how it is possible to realise it if you stick around to find out what could happen. Turn some of that suicidal energy towards risking change in your life. Consider that it may be a behaviour pattern or life condition that you want to end. Ask yourself, "What inside me needs to die?"

Some ideas for good self-care:

1. **Embodying practices**: Sometimes, our mental chatter can be overbearing and make us feel heavy and overwhelmed. Embodying practices, such as exercise, movement, mindfulness and BREATHING, not only bring us into the present moment, but give us a chance to create space between thoughts.

2. **Create a sacred space**, be it a place where you keep things that are meaningful to you, or a room that is your safe haven and your chance to reconnect with yourself.

3. **Spend time in nature**, whether it's by the sea, a woodland, or even just some fresh air outside your house or your office, spending time in the natural world not only brings us freedom but can reconnect us to our presence, our aliveness.

4. **Practice Gratitude**. However hard it may be, try to take a moment to look at all the things you have to be thankful for in your life. Be grateful for the smallest of things, maybe things you take for granted. Be grateful for your bed? Maybe that you have a roof over your head? Maybe you have access to food and clean water? Starting small and working up, inviting more gratitude into your life can transform the way you see and show up in life. This is scientifically proven to rewire our brain.

5. **Build up your inner wellspring of self-worth.** Whether it be writing down an affirmation and sticking it to your bathroom mirror, creating an empowering and uplifting mantra to chant to yourself every morning, surrounding yourself with people who remind you of your innate worthiness, smiling at yourself when you catch your reflection, listening to uplifting music that makes you feel powerful and ready to take on the world, becoming aware of those inner critics that try to keep you small...whatever it may be, try to create a life that reflects your innate worthiness back to you. Your self-worth does NOT depend on what your profession might or might not be, it doesn't depend on how much you please other people...it is innately yours and it is already within you.

6. **Become aware of what's energising you** and what is draining you. Say YES to the things that energise and nurture you and NO to the things that drain your energy or no longer serve you. Set boundaries! This is easier said than done sometimes, we highly recommend *Braving the Wilderness* by Brené Brown for guidance on setting healthy boundaries.

7. **Thank Your Body** for all the things it does for you every second of every day. While you are reading this, your heart is pumping, your lungs are breathing, your digestive system is working to turn the food you ate earlier into energy, your cells are being healed and renewed. There are

thousands of biochemical reactions happening that we have no say in, our body does that on its own. Let's thank it for what it does for us and allows us to do.

8. **Read.** Take a look at our recommended reading list in the Resources section of this book for some empowering and life-changing reading.

9. **Create with your heart.** Creativity can come in as many different forms as there are people in this world, whether it's writing, painting, sculpting, singing…tap into those creative juices running through you. Try focusing on the process of creating as opposed to the end product…get messy, have a play and tap into your inner child.

10. **Trust the healing process.** The road to recovery is not always a linear one, sometimes it's a case of taking one step forward and two steps back and that's okay.

11. **Connect with supportive and inspiring people**, who are willing to listen without judgement and an open heart. If you can't find them in person, join an online group.

12. **Find a safe space** to be vulnerable, to speak your truth, express your feelings. Maybe with a therapist or a mentor.

13. **Join a support group**. Connect with people who are going through similar things and build each other up.

14. **Diversify your social media feed.** All day, every day we are bombarded with messages from different kinds of screens. Taking control of what we are exposed to can drastically improve our mental health and wellbeing. Choosing to see more positive posts will not only allow your brain to create new neural pathways and create a new 'normal', but you will feel more uplifted and at peace with yourself.

15. **Celebrate every success**. Sometimes all these things can seem too much or even unimaginable to do. Sometimes self-care comes in the form of getting out of bed in the morning, cleaning your teeth, having a wash...Give yourself a pat on the back and celebrate every success you can. You are doing an amazing job and we are so proud of you for not giving up!

You can do this!

Glossary

Alhumdulillah – Arabic phrase meaning "All thanks be to God"

Alhumdulillah ala Kulli haal – Praise be to God in every circumstance.

Allah (SWT) – is the Arabic term for God.

Allah's messenger or Rasul Allah – refers to the Prophet Muhammad (SAW) born in Arabia approximately 1400 years ago.

Ayah – verses from the Quran.

Bismillah ir Rahman ir Raheem – In the name of God, the Most Gracious, the Most Merciful.

Dhikr – is a prayer or an act of remembering God.

Duaa – Invocation an act of supplication/prayer, worship, to "call out" and Muslims regard this as a profound act of worship.

Evil Eye – a form of intense jealousy from one person to another that can have negative implications on one's life

Fitra – A natural connection to God (Allah) which Muslims believe all humans are born with.

Hadith – or a tradition is saying ascribed to the Prophet Muhammad (Pbuh).

Hikmah – Arabic meaning wisdom, philosophy; rationale, underlying reason.

In sha' Allah – means 'God willing' is used when speaking about future events whose outcome is determined by God.

Islam – is the religion Muslims believe was revealed to the Prophet Muhammad (saw) in Arabia at the beginning of the 7th century. Islam literally means 'submission to the will of God'. For Muslims, Islam represents a return to the monotheistic faith of the Prophet Abraham and recognises Moses and Jesus as prophets.

Jinn – Another type of being created by God alongside humans and angels

Mash'Allah – God has willed it; an expression of gratitude.

Muslim – one who practices Islam.

Nafs – The human soul or 'self'

Pbuh – Peace and blessings be upon him (This expression follows after mentioning the name of the Prophet Muhammad.

Qadar – Arabic meaning "fate" divine fore-ordainment, predestination.

Qalb – Spiritual heart that resides in the physical heart and is the centre for consciousness, thought, reasoning, intentions and connection to God

Qur'an – The book Muslims believe was revealed by God (Allah) through the angel Gabriel to the Prophet Muhammad (SAW).

Ramadan – is the month in the Arabic calendar when Muslims fast during daylight hours and is one of the five pillars of faith.

Raqi – Spiritual Healer (according to some Muslim communities)

Ruh – Spirit or Life force

Ruqya – Spiritual healing (according to the Qur'an and Sunnah)

Sabr – Patience

SAW – is an acronym of *Sall Allahu alay-hi wa-sallam in Arabic* meaning ' Peace and blessings be upon him' in Arabic, and follows any mention of the Prophet Muhammad.

Shahada – or bearing witness, is the first pillar of the five Islamic pillars and a declaration of faith. *La ilaha ilalla wa Muahmmad ur-rasul Allah*, which means 'There is no true God but God and Muhammad is his messenger'.

Shirk – Arabic – idolatry, polytheism, and the association of God with other deities.

Sihr – is what magicians do to cause delusion, death, sickness, separation between husband and wife and many other kinds of harm to people through tying knots or shayateen (devils) or Jinn. All sihr is forbidden in Islam.

SWT – is an acronym of *Subhanahu Wa Ta'ala*, meaning 'May He be glorified and exalted', and follows any mention of Allah, God.

Sunnah – Sayings and practices of the prophet Muhammad.

Surah – a chapter of the Quran.

Taqwa – means awareness or mindfulness of Allah (SWT).

Tawakkul – Reliance of God – trusting in God's plan.

Ummah – can mean the community or nation of Muslims, or sometimes humanity as a whole.

Acknowledgements

My (Katie) infinite thanks go to the incredible Kinda Proud team; the book Reps, and especially Ayan Hussein, Sophia and Sara for spearheading this particular edition in the series. All of whom have passionately, and without question, donated their time and expertise in order to support this project to fruition. It's a vision we all share, and one that would not have been possible to achieve without each and every one of us coming together with no agenda other than wanting to disseminate hope like confetti around the world...

The 'Muslim Emerging Proud Team' would like to thank Allah (subhanahu wataallah) for making this possible, guiding us, healing us, loving us, and being an eternal source of Hope. We would also like to extend our immense gratitude to everyone in this pocket book, who have bravely given their personal transformation story with the hope that it helps at least one other person in the world to find their own inner spark to initiate or aid their recovery journey. We aim for these books to create a 'positive domino effect', rippling out HOPE to those who need it most.

Without all of these team players there would be no HOPE confetti, so together we celebrate the incredible power of heart-founded collaboration, and a shared vision and mission.

We would also like to thank the people who funded this book and made it possible who would like to remain anonymous.

Other titles in our Kinda Proud Pocket Books of Hope and Transformation series so far:

#Emerging Proud through NOTEs (non-ordinary transcendent experiences)

#Emerging Proud through Disordered Eating, Body Image and Low Self-Esteem

#Emerging Proud through Suicide

#Emerging Proud through Trauma and Abuse

Eye Inspire: #Emerging Proud through Eye Sight Loss

> *"For indeed, with hardship [will be] ease.*
> *Indeed, with hardship [will be] ease."*
>
> Qur'an Surah Ash-Shar, 94:5-6

Surah al-Inshirah, meaning "Solace" or "Comfort", is the 94th Surah of The Quran. It is also known as Surah ash-Sharh, literally, "The Opening-up of the Heart".

As the name suggests, Surah al-Inshirah thematically deals with comforting and offering solace to believers. It is believed to have been revealed in Mecca, during the early days of Islam — that was a period of great difficulty, as people were still hostile to the Message of Islam, and to Prophet Muhammad (PBUH) in particular. As such, Surah al-Inshirah came as a Word of Encouragement from Allah (SWT) to the Prophet (PBUH) and his Ummah.

This Surah repeats the verse "Verily, with hardship, comes ease." twice, effectively implying that for each difficulty faced by us, Allah sends us twice the relief or reward.

Surah al-Inshirah: Peace and Solace for Troubled Hearts | Quranic Quotes; https://quranicquotes. com/notes/surah-inshirah/

Hope

It's all I need

to lift my heart

out of the depths

and into the light

— Ambriel

Our team

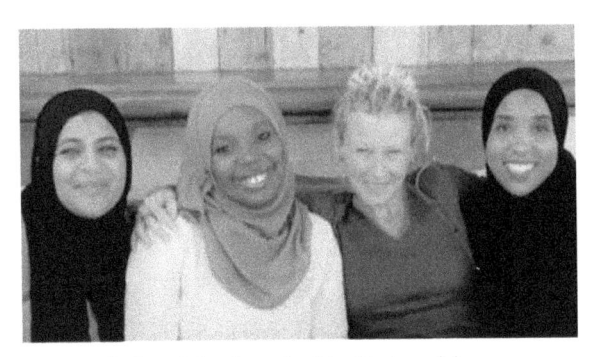

Left to right: Sara, Sophia, Katie and Ayan

Working with the Muslim team on this book has been such an honour and a privilege. I have learned and grown so much throughout the process thanks to these inspiring women. We may have different views of 'faith', but we connect deeply in shared values and real human emotions – these are where bridges are built and any differences pale into insignificance. Long live real, authentic heart connections. **Katie, Publisher**

I would like to express my deepest gratitude to Katie and the Muslim team Sophia and Sara, for all your help, support and friendship throughout the book's journey. It has been an incredible journey, full of learning and growing. You guys made the work feel a lot easier. It is truly a blessing to witness the book coming together. I hope and pray that this book inspires and touches many souls and creates HOPE. I have come to learn that we may have our differences in race, culture or 'faith'. However, we share commonalities such as human behaviours, emotions and feelings. Therefore, to find unity in diversity, we need to recognise our differences, not just our similarities, and celebrate them in all people. **Ayan Hussein, Rep**

Contact the team via their new organisation:

Chapters of Solace - A supportive space for Muslims going through Mental Distress

www.chaptersofsolace.com